Map Key

Trail Name

DAY & OVERNIGHT HIKES

Anza-Borrego Desert

STATE PARK

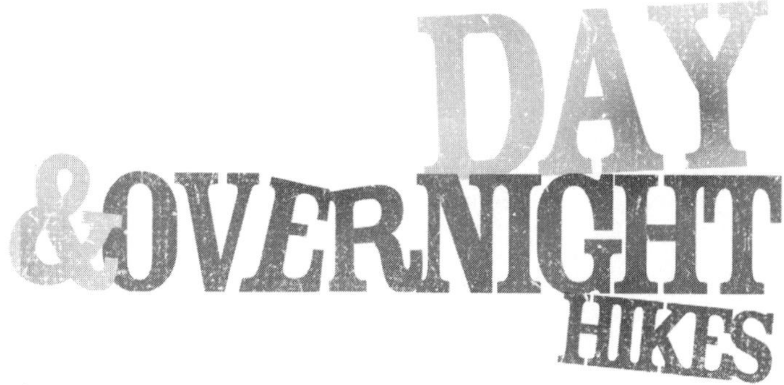

Anza-Borrego Desert

STATE PARK

Sheri McGregor

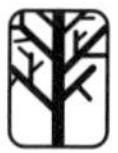

Menasha Ridge Press

DISCLAIMER

This book is meant only as a guide to select trails within Anza-Borrego Desert State Park and does not guarantee hiker safety in any way—you hike at your own risk. Neither Menasha Ridge Press nor Sheri McGregor is liable for property loss or damage, personal injury, or death that result in any way from accessing or hiking the trails described in the following pages. Please be aware that hikers have been injured and that hiker deaths have occurred in the Anza-Borrego Desert State Park region. Be especially cautious when walking on or near boulders, steep inclines, and drop-offs, and do not attempt to explore terrain that may be beyond your abilities. To help ensure an uneventful hike, please read carefully the introduction to this book, and perhaps get further safety information and guidance from the park directly. Familiarize yourself thoroughly with the areas you intend to visit before venturing out. Ask questions, and prepare for the unforeseen. Familiarize yourself with current weather reports, maps of the area you intend to visit, and park regulations.

Printed in the United States of America
Published by Menasha Ridge Press
Distributed by The Globe Pequot Press
First edition, first printing

Cover and text design by Ian Szymkowiak, Palace Press International, Inc.
Cover photo by Karl Weatherly © Getty Images
Author photo by William Kordela
Maps by Scott McGrew, Steve Jones, and Sheri McGregor

Library of Congress Cataloging-in-Publication Data

McGregor, Sheri, 1961–
Day and overnight hikes in Anza-Borrego Desert State Park/by Sheri McGregor.
p. cm.
Includes index.
ISBN 13: 978-0-89732-971-2
ISBN 10: 0-89732-971-6

1. Hiking—California—Anza-Borrego Desert State Park—Guidebooks. 2. Anza-Borrego Desert State Park (Calif.)—Guidebooks. I. Title.

GV199.42.C2M345 2006
917.54'85—dc22

2006047258

Menasha Ridge Press
P.O. Box 43673
Birmingham, AL 35243
www.menasharidge.com

Table of Contents

Dedication

*To those who walk in nature and find themselves at home—
enjoy!*

Acknowledgments

Biggest thanks go to Brian McGregor whose relentless "mission" pushed me to keep up, but who also always waited (somewhere!) on the path ahead while I communed with tiny, magnificent wonders. I would also like to acknowledge Diana and Lowell Lindsay, whose *Anza-Borrego Desert Region* map I recommend for anyone trekking into the area.

Preface

WITH MORE THAN 600,000 ACRES OF OPEN SPACE, Anza-Borrego Desert State Park is a world of wonders. While mostly within San Diego County, California, the park also stretches north into Riverside County, east into Imperial County, and nearly into Mexico at its southernmost point. Many consider the desert dry and desolate, but secret oases, cool waterfalls, interesting animals, and a wide array of adaptive vegetation wait quietly to refresh adventurous souls.

Those seeking solitude can find it here in the largest desert state park in the contiguous United States. More-sociable types also enjoy this recreational mecca, which includes ample four-wheel-drive and off-road access areas, equestrian and hiking trails, and plentiful camping opportunities.

One developed campground, Tamarisk Grove, offers full hookups, tent sites, restrooms and showers, and a variety of activities. Similar facilities are available on the grounds of Agua Caliente, a full-service county park within the state park.

Other established sites feature a more primitive camping experience. Popular dry camps include Blair Valley, Bow Willow, Culp Valley, Fish Creek, Mountain Palm Springs, and Sheep Canyon. Some of these sites do have chemical toilets, shade ramadas, and picnic tables. Note that only Bow Willow has trashcans.

Besides the officially established sites, Anza-Borrego Desert State Park has an "open camping" policy—meaning you can pack in supplies and camp almost anywhere, taking care to obey closure signs and keep off any private property. Bring your own firewood, pack in a fireproof metal container to completely contain your fire, and be sure to keep flames and smoke to a minimum so you don't damage or discolor anything in the park. To cook, you must use a portable stove. And don't forget to pack out anything you bring in or create on site. Leave no trash, ashes, or debris of any kind behind.

Some sites in Anza-Borrego Desert State Park require fees for day or overnight use. I've noted this at individual trails, but rules and requirements change. You'll see posted signs indicating that visitors are expected to know the rules, so get them at the Visitor Center, 200 Palm Canyon Drive, Borrego Springs, or phone the park for information, (760) 767-5311.

Whether you day-hike or you like to get closer to the desert by backpacking and camping in the park, leave your worries at the gate and allow the desert's natural features to serenade you. Nature's melody may come to you in a classic call of the wild, like the haunting cries of coyotes yipping in the night, or it may be even more forceful, like the buffeting rhythm of strong desert wind whistling through boulder stands, up over hills, into valleys, and whipping at your hair and clothes. But nature also sings more-subtle songs—like the melody found in the gentle swish of an ocotillo's spindly bloom-tipped arms, the promised explosion of color resting within a cactus bloom's curled bud, or the whisper-soft caress of an arid desert breeze.

As scorching heat is swallowed in a twilight-pink sky, hungry bats awaken and emerge on nimble wings, a restless predator rises to prowl, and stars grow bright. At dawn, the powdery sand is moist with dew, holding the scuttling imprints of tiny insects that scurried in the night. A tarantula hawk flits about on transparent red wings. A dragonfly hovers, beckoning you to a stream's edge where water splashes, sprays, and tumbles, reflecting the lilting dance of your soul awakened by the desert.

Hiking Recommendations

Most Scenic Hikes

2 Hellhole Canyon to Maidenhair Falls (page 28)
6 Borrego Palm Canyon to South Fork Falls (page 46)
9 Cougar Canyon (page 65)
13 Butler Canyon–Rockhouse Canyon Loop (page 85)
15 Whale Peak (page 97)
17 Oriflamme Canyon (page 105)
31 South Carrizo Creek–Canyon Sin Nombre Loop (page 171)

Most Difficult Hikes

3 Flat Cat Canyon (page 33)
4 California Riding and Hiking Trail (page 38)
6 Borrego Palm Canyon to South Fork Falls (page 46)
8 Sheep Canyon (page 60)
9 Cougar Canyon (page 65)
17 Oriflamme Canyon (page 105)

Easiest Hikes

5 Borrego Palm Canyon Nature Trail (page 42)
18 The Mortreros (page 111)
19 Pictograph Trail (page 113)
24 Elephant Trees Nature Loop (page 140)
27 Mud Hills Wash to Elephant Knees (page 150)
28 San Sebastian Marsh (page 154)
29 Moonlight Canyon Loop (page 161)

Best-maintained Trails

5 Borrego Palm Canyon Nature Trail (page 42)
19 Pictograph Trail (page 113)
20 Ghost Mountain (page 116)
29 Moonlight Canyon Loop (page 161)

Best Hikes for Solitude

9 Cougar Canyon (page 65)
10 Indian Canyon (page 71)
11 Horse Canyon (page 74)
12 White Wash (page 78)
13 Butler Canyon–Rockhouse Canyon Loop (page 85)
15 Whale Peak (page 97)
16 Rainbow Canyon Loop (page 102)
21 Bow Willow–Rockhouse Canyon Loop (page 124)
25 Alma Wash (page 144)

Best Hikes for Children

2 Hellhole Canyon to Maidenhair Falls (page 28)
5 Borrego Palm Canyon Nature Trail (page 42)

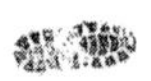

19 Pictograph Trail (page 113)
20 Ghost Mountain (page 116)
24 Elephant Trees Nature Loop (page 140)

Best Hikes for Wildflowers

1 Wilson Trail (page 24)
2 Hellhole Canyon to Maidenhair Falls (page 28)
4 California Riding and Hiking Trail (page 38)
5 Borrego Palm Canyon Nature Trail (page 42)
16 Rainbow Canyon Loop (page 102)
17 Oriflamme Canyon (page 105)
21 Bow Willow–Rockhouse Canyon Loop (page 124)
22 Mountain Palm Springs Loop (page 128)

Best Hikes for Wildlife

3 Flat Cat Canyon (page 33)
4 California Riding and Hiking Trail (page 38)
5 Borrego Palm Canyon Nature Trail (page 42)
9 Cougar Canyon (page 65)
10 Indian Canyon (page 71)
11 Horse Canyon (page 74)
12 White Wash (page 78)

Hikes with Dogs

Dogs are not allowed on nature trails

Wheelchair-accessible Hikes

None

Steep Hikes

3 Flat Cat Canyon (page 33)
4 California Riding and Hiking Trail (page 38)
8 Sheep Canyon (page 60)
9 Cougar Canyon (page 65)
14 Pinyon Mountain (page 94)
15 Whale Peak (page 97)
20 Ghost Mountain (page 116)
26 Wind Caves Loop (page 147)

Flat (or Mostly Flat) Hikes

1 Wilson Trail (page 24)
2 Hellhole Canyon to Maidenhair Falls (page 28)
5 Borrego Palm Canyon Nature Trail (page 42)
10 Indian Canyon (page 71)
11 Horse Canyon (page 74)
18 The Mortreros (page 111)
24 Elephant Trees Nature Loop (page 140)

Hiking Recommendations *(continued)*

Flat (or Mostly Flat) Hikes (continued)

Hikes with Historical Points of Interest

Introduction

THE NAME ANZA-BORREGO combines an important historical figure and the desert wilderness that still exists today. *Anza* refers to Juan Bautista de Anza, whose expeditions opened the first roadway into California. *Borrego* is the Spanish word for "lamb"—fitting because the region is home to wild Peninsular bighorn sheep. In essence, the life and journeys of de Anza provide a metaphor for the idea of progress and the settling of lands. The Peninsular bighorn sheep, now endangered, represent the wild. Thus, the joining of these two words demonstrates the delicate balance between civilization and wilderness, which is well presented in Anza-Borrego Desert State Park. While the park is open to visitors, some areas are subject to a few months' annual closure to protect the sheep's water sources, so the struggle continues to preserve the land while allowing human enjoyment. Continued reevaluation sometimes results in change. As recently as 2005, a large portion of park acreage was permanently closed to vehicle traffic to protect natural habitat. Foot travel is still allowed and, with respect and care by visitors, will continue.

As hikers, we appreciate our parklands as a valuable resource, and we strive to honor the delicate balance between ourselves and nature.

How to Use This Guidebook

The Overview Map and Overview-map Key

Use the overview map on the inside front cover to assess the location of each hike's primary trailhead. Each hike's number appears on the overview map, on the map key facing the overview map, and in the table of contents.

Trail Maps

Each hike contains a detailed map that shows the trailhead, the route, significant features, facilities, and topographic landmarks such as creeks, overlooks, and peaks. The author gathered map data by carrying a Garmin Etrex GPS unit while hiking. This data was downloaded into DeLorme's TopoUSA digital mapping program and then processed by expert cartographers to produce the highly accurate maps found in this book.

Elevation Profiles

Corresponding directly to the trail map, each hike contains a detailed elevation profile. The elevation profile provides a quick look at the trail from the side, enabling you to visualize how the trail rises and falls. Note the number of feet between each tick mark on the vertical axis (the height scale). To avoid making flat hikes look steep and steep hikes appear flat, appropriate height scales are used throughout the book to provide an accurate image of the hike's climbing difficulty. Elevation profiles for loop hikes show total distance; those for out-and-back hikes show only one-way distance.

GPS Trailhead Coordinates

To collect accurate map data, the author hiked each trail with a handheld Garmin Etrex GPS unit. Data collected was then downloaded and plotted onto a digital U.S. Geological Survey–based topographic map. In addition to rendering a highly specific trail outline, this book also includes the GPS coordinates for each trailhead in two formats: latitude–longitude and UTM (Universal Transverse Mercator). Latitude–longitude coordinates employ a grid system that indicates your location by crossroading a line that runs north to south with a line that runs east to west. Lines of latitude are parallel and run east to west. The 0° line of latitude is the equator. Lines of longitude are not parallel, run north to south, and converge at the North and South poles. The 0° line of longitude passes through Greenwich, England.

Topographic maps show latitude and longitude as well as UTM grid lines. Known as UTM coordinates, the numbers index a specific point, also using a grid method. The survey information, or datum, used to arrive at the coordinates in this book is WGS84 (versus NAD27 or WGS83). For readers who own a GPS unit, whether handheld or onboard a vehicle, the latitude–longitude or UTM coordinates provided on the first page of each hike may be entered into the GPS unit. Just make sure your GPS unit is set to navigate using WGS84 datum. Now you can navigate directly to the trailhead.

Trailheads in parking areas can be reached by car, but some hikes still require a short walk to reach the trailhead from the parking area. In those cases, a handheld unit is necessary to continue the GPS navigation process. That said, readers can easily access all trailheads in this book by using the directions given, the overview map, and the trail map, which shows at least one significant road leading into the area. But for those who enjoy using the latest GPS technology to navigate, the necessary data has been provided. A brief explanation of the UTM coordinates for Rainbow Canyon Loop (page 102) follows.

UTM Zone	11S
Easting	550780
Northing	3652244

The UTM zone number 11 refers to one of the 60 vertical zones of the UTM projection, each of which is 6 degrees wide. *S* refers to horizontal zones, each of which is 8 degrees wide except for Zone X (12 degrees wide). The easting number 550780 indicates in meters how far east or west a point is from the central meridian of the zone. Increasing easting coordinates on a topographic map or on your GPS screen indicate that you are moving east; decreasing easting coordinates indicate that you are moving west. The northing number 3652244 references in meters how far you are from the equator.

Increasing northing coordinates indicate you are traveling north; decreasing northing coordinates indicate you are traveling south. To learn more about how to enhance your outdoor experiences with GPS technology, refer to *GPS Outdoors: A Practical Guide for Outdoor Enthusiasts* (Menasha Ridge Press).

The Hike Profile

In addition to maps, each hike contains a concise but informative narrative of the hike from beginning to end. Within the text you'll find common hiking terms such as "rock ducks" or "cairns"—the small stacks of rocks left by other hikers to help mark the route. This descriptive text is enhanced with at-a-glance ratings and information, GPS-based trailhead coordinates, and accurate driving directions that lead you from a major road to the parking area most convenient to the trailhead.

At the top of the section for each hike is a box that allows the hiker quick access to pertinent information: quality of scenery, condition of trail, appropriateness for children, difficulty of hike, quality of solitude expected, hike distance, approximate time of hike, and outstanding highlights of the trip. The first five categories are rated using a five-star system. On the next page is an example.

The two stars indicate the scenery is somewhat picturesque. The three stars following indicate it is a moderately easy hike (five stars for difficulty would be strenuous). The four stars mean that the trail condition is very good (one star would mean the trail is likely to be muddy, rocky, overgrown, or otherwise compromised). The five stars for solitude mean you can expect to encounter only a few people on the trail (with one star you may well be elbowing your way up the trail). And the final three stars indicate that the hike is doable for able-bodied children (a one-star rating would denote that only the most gung-ho and physically fit children should go).

Distances given are absolute, but hiking times are estimated for an average hiking speed of 2 to 3 miles per hour, with time

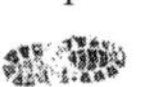

1 Wilson Trail

SCENERY: ☆☆
DIFFICULTY: ☆☆☆
TRAIL CONDITION: ☆☆☆☆
SOLITUDE: ☆☆☆☆☆
CHILDREN: ☆☆☆
DISTANCE: *8.7 miles round trip*
HIKING TIME: *4–5 hours*
OUTSTANDING FEATURES: *Predominantly flat with some hills and dales, wildflowers in spring, horned lizards, rock formations, view of the desert valley and the Salton Sea*

built in for pauses at overlooks and brief rests. Naturally, if you backpack in and stay overnight, you will need to adjust those times accordingly.

Following each box is a brief italicized description of the hike. A more detailed account follows in which elements such as trail junctions, stream crossings, and trailside features are noted, along with their distance from the trailhead. Flip through the book, read the descriptions, choose a hike that appeals to you, and prepare for it accordingly.

Weather

Each of the four seasons occurs in Anza-Borrego Desert State Park, with snow sometimes falling when it's cold enough in the higher elevations, and spring showers bringing beautiful flowers. Of course, heat is what people typically associate with the desert—and it *does* get hot. Don't hike in the summer months, when temperatures routinely exceed 100°F. Also, be aware that flash floods, electrical storms, and dangerous winds are possible year-round. Know the expected weather before you go, and watch for changes. Even on moderate days in fall or spring, you'll need to wear layered clothing as a safeguard. The temperature inside a canyon or within the walls of a gorge can dip much lower than that on an open trail in full sun.

The average-temperature chart below refers to temperatures in Borrego Springs. As noted above, temperatures within different areas of the park itself can vary considerably, dipping well below or above those reflected in the chart. (According to locals, you can predict the high temperature for the day by taking the morning low and adding 30 degrees.)

Average Temperature by Month (Fahrenheit)

	Jan	Feb	Mar	Apr	May	Jun
High	69	73	77	84	93	102
Low	58	43	49	53	60	68
	Jul	Aug	Sep	Oct	Nov	Dec
High	107	105	100	90	78	69
Low	75	74	69	60	50	43

In general, the desert recreational season begins in October, when the highs begin tapering down to double digits, and the lows are at or above 60. These temperatures make backpacking enjoyable in the fall. By winter, you'll want to rethink tent camping, although with the right equipment, temperatures dipping into the low 40s at night are still manageable. By March, average nighttime temperatures begin to climb a little, and the days are also fairly mild, making this one of the most popular months for camping. April and May are still fairly mild but variable. And no matter what month you go, as mentioned above, be aware of impending storms and prepare for weather variations. Those who have spent time in the sometimes-unforgiving wilderness know that it's better to overprepare than be caught off guard. Each year brings news of people who become lost or get caught unprepared in a storm. Injuries, heat stroke, and deaths do occur. Be prepared, avoid taking risks, and you won't be another statistic.

Water

How much is enough? Well, one simple physiological fact should convince you to err on the side of excess when deciding how much water to pack: A hiker working hard in 90-degree heat needs about 10 quarts of fluid per day. That's 2.5 gallons—12 large water bottles or 16 small ones. In other words, pack along one or two bottles even for short hikes.

Most of the water sources described in this book cannot be considered reliable. Only a few specific desert areas boast water flow all year-round, so don't count on the presence of water. Simply put, not bringing an adequate water supply with you into the desert is foolhardy.

Even where water is perennial as noted herein, choosing to drink it comes with risks. Some hikers and backpackers are prepared to purify water found along the route. But even this method, while less dangerous than drinking it untreated, can be dangerous. Purifiers with ceramic filters are the safest. Many hikers pack along the slightly distasteful tetraglycine-hydroperiodide tablets to debug water (sold under names such as Potable Aqua and Coughlan's).

Probably the most common waterborne "bug" that hikers face is giardia, which may not hit until one to four weeks after ingestion. It will have you living in the bathroom, passing noxious rotten-egg gas, vomiting, and shivering with chills. Other parasites to worry about include E. coli and cryptosporidium, both of which are harder to kill than giardia.

For most people, the pleasures of hiking make carrying water a relatively minor price to pay to remain healthy. If you're tempted to drink found water, you should do so only if you understand the risks involved. Better yet, hydrate prior to your hike, carry (and drink) eight ounces of water for every mile you plan to hike, and hydrate after the hike.

Clothing

There is a wide variety of clothing from which to choose. Be prepared for anything. If all you have are cotton clothes when a sudden rainstorm comes along, you'll be miserable, especially in cooler weather. It's a good idea to carry along a light wool sweater or some type of synthetic apparel (polypropylene, Capilene, Thermax, or the like) and wear a wide-brimmed sun-protection hat. A hat with a flap that can be fastened up or let down to cover your neck keeps you protected as the sun travels across the sky.

Although rain gear is available and a good idea for those hiking in wet weather, I don't recommend hiking in desert storms. The elements can be disorienting, flash floods can occur, and strong winds can rip even the hardiest of hikers off their feet.

Footwear is another concern. Desert trails can be slippery, rocky, and studded with nasty thorns. Waterproofed or not, hiking boots should be your footwear of choice. Ankle-high styles offer more protection against spiky vegetation and also provide more support. Sport sandals are popular, but they leave much of your foot exposed and therefore aren't appropriate for desert hiking. An injured foot far from the trailhead can make for a miserable limp back to the car. Ditto for wet feet, so consult the individual hike write-ups, and consider waterproof boots.

The Essentials

One of the first rules of hiking is to be prepared for anything. The simplest way to be prepared is to carry the essentials. In addition to carrying the items listed on the next page, you need to know how to use them, especially the navigation items. Always consider worst-case scenarios such as getting lost, hiking back in the dark, broken gear (say, a broken hip strap on your pack or a water filter getting plugged), twisting an ankle, or a brutal thunderstorm. The items listed below don't cost a lot of money, don't take up much room in a pack, and don't weigh much—but they might just save your life.

WATER: durable bottles and water treatment such as iodine or a filter

MAP: preferably a topo map and a trail map with a route description. I also recommend Diana and Lowell Lindsay's *Anza-Borrego Desert Region* map for anyone trekking into the area.

COMPASS

MIRROR: this will help attract attention from airplanes in emergencies

BANDANA: another attention-getter (tie to the top of a creosote tree)

FIRST-AID KIT: a good-quality kit including first-aid instructions

KNIFE: a multitool device with pliers is best

LIGHT: flashlight or headlamp with extra bulbs and batteries

FIRE: windproof matches or lighter and fire starter

EXTRA FOOD: you should always have some left when you've finished hiking

EXTRA CLOTHES: rain protection, warm layers, gloves, warm hat

SUN PROTECTION: sunglasses, lip balm, sunblock, sun hat

OTHER ITEMS I OFTEN CARRY INTO THE DESERT:

A lightweight thermal blanket (a foil one is ideal)

A roll of duct tape

Rope (professional-grade rappelling rope is best)

First-aid Kit

A typical first-aid kit may contain more items than you might think necessary. The ones on the following page are just the basics. Prepackaged kits in waterproof bags (Atwater Carey and Adventure Medical make a variety of kits) are available. Though there are quite a few items listed here, they pack into a small space:

- Ace bandages or Spenco joint wraps
- Antibiotic ointment (Neosporin or the generic equivalent)
- Aspirin or acetaminophen
- Band-Aids
- Benadryl or its generic equivalent, diphenhydramine (in case of allergic reactions)
- Butterfly-closure bandages
- Epinephrine in a prefilled syringe (for severe allergic reactions)
- Gauze (one roll)
- Gauze compress pads (a half-dozen 4- by 4-inch pads)
- Hydrogen peroxide or iodine
- Insect repellent
- Matches or pocket lighter
- Moleskin or Spenco Second Skin
- Sunscreen
- Whistle (it's more effective than your voice in signaling rescuers because it doesn't sound natural and is loud)

Hiking with Children

No one is too young for a hike, but take special care in the desert, with its cacti, other thorny plants, and severe weather. Most of the hikes in this book simply aren't suitable for children. Fit children older than age 10 may be able to handle flat, short trails, but the lack of shade, remote location, and unforgiving climate make hiking with toddlers and infants inappropriate. Use common sense to judge a child's capacity to hike a particular trail. A list of hikes that are suitable for children is provided on page xiv. Do read the individual write-ups even for those hikes, though. Then consider your own child's abilities when making a decision.

General Safety

The desert can be a barren, dangerous place, but to those who take the time to prepare and explore this vast wilderness, the area reveals its natural treasure. Potentially dangerous situations can occur, but preparation and sound judgment result in safe forays into the remote desert. Here are a few tips to make your trip safer and easier.

- **ALWAYS CARRY FOOD AND WATER,** whether you are planning an overnight trip or not. Food will give you energy, help keep you warm, and sustain you in an emergency situation until help arrives. You never know if you will have a stream nearby when you become thirsty. Bring potable water, or boil/filter water before drinking it from a stream.
- **WEAR STURDY SHOES,** along with a hat and plenty of sunscreen.
- **NEVER HIKE ALONE**—take a buddy with you out on the trails.
- **TELL SOMEONE WHERE YOU'RE GOING** and when you'll be back (be as specific as possible), and ask him or her to get help if you don't return in a reasonable amount of time.
- **STAY ON THE TRAILS AND ROUTES DESCRIBED HEREIN.** Most hikers get lost when they leave the path. Even on the most clearly marked trails, there is usually a point where you have to stop and consider which direction to head. If you become disoriented, don't panic. As soon as you think you may be off track, stop, assess your current direction, and then retrace your steps back to the point where you went awry. Using a map, a compass, and this book, and keeping in mind what you have passed thus far, reorient yourself and trust your judgment on which way to continue. If you become absolutely unsure of how to proceed, return to your vehicle the way you came in. Should you become completely lost and have no idea of how to return to the trailhead, remaining in place along the trail and waiting for help is most often the best choice for adults and always the best option for children. If you have prepared well, brought supplies, and taken that all-important step of telling someone where you'll be and for how long, staying in place won't result in disaster.
- **BE ESPECIALLY CAREFUL WHEN CROSSING STREAMS.** Whether you are fording a stream or crossing on a log or rocks, watch every step.
- **MAKE SURE YOUR CAR, TRUCK, OR SUV** is in good shape before you go to the park, and check road conditions before you set out. If your vehicle breaks down, stay with it—it's easier to find a vehicle than a person.
- **WHEN CLIMBING OVER BOULDERS,** be careful where you put your hands. Be aware of the possibility of snakes. When you are climbing down big boulders, make sure you're not sliding into an area you can't

climb back out of (bring rope, and never hike alone). Also, when moving over boulders, be aware that some may be loose, so tread carefully. And what looks like solid ground might just be clumped mud, meaning your foot will slip through to nothing underneath.

- **BE CAREFUL AT OVERLOOKS.** While these areas may provide spectacular views, they are potentially hazardous. Stay back from the edge of outcrops and be absolutely sure of your footing; a misstep can mean a nasty and possibly fatal fall.
- **STANDING DEAD TREES AND STORM-DAMAGED LIVING TREES** pose a real hazard to hikers and tent campers. These trees may have loose or broken limbs that could fall at any time. When choosing a spot to rest or a backcountry campsite, look up. When hiking through woody areas, be careful not to hook your pack or clothing on a stray limb. Getting "hooked" can throw you off balance and cause injury.
- **KNOW THE SYMPTOMS OF HEAT-RELATED EMERGENCIES,** and prevent dehydration (drink water even before you are thirsty). There are three heat emergencies you should be aware of and know how to handle:

  Heat cramps—painful cramps in the leg and abdomen, along with excessive sweating and feeling faint. Caused by the body's loss of too much salt, heat cramps must be handled by getting to a cool place and sipping water or an electrolyte solution.

  Heat exhaustion—dizziness, headache, irregular pulse, disorientation, and nausea are all symptoms of heat exhaustion, which occurs as blood vessels dilate and attempt to move heat from the inner body to the skin. Get to a cool place and drink cool water. Get a buddy to fan you, which can help cool you off more quickly.

  Heatstroke—dilated pupils; dry, hot, flushed skin; a rapid pulse; high fever; and abnormal breathing are all symptoms of heatstroke, a life-threatening condition that can cause convulsions, unconsciousness, or even death. If you think a hiking partner is experiencing heatstroke, get him or her to a cool place and find help. (*Note:* Cell phones very rarely work in the park—you might find reception in spots near the main roads, but even then it's not reliable.)
- **KNOW THE SYMPTOMS OF HYPOTHERMIA,** or subnormal body temperature. Shivering and forgetfulness are the two most common indicators of this insidious killer. Hypothermia can occur at any elevation, even

in summer, especially when the hiker is wearing lightweight cotton clothing. If symptoms arise, give the victim shelter, hot liquids, and dry clothes or a dry sleeping bag.

- **TAKE ALONG YOUR BRAIN.** A cool, calculating mind is the single most important piece of equipment you'll need on the trail. Think before you act. Watch your step. Plan ahead. Avoiding accidents before they happen is the best recipe for a rewarding and relaxing hike.
- **ASK QUESTIONS.** Park rangers are there to help. It's a lot easier to get advice beforehand and avoid mishaps away from civilization, where finding help may be difficult. Use your head out there and treat the place as if it were your own backyard. After all, it is your state park.

Animal and Plant Hazards

Ticks

Ticks are commonly found in brush and woody areas. Therefore, you are less likely to encounter them in desert areas than in other regions. Some hikes, though, do go through wooded areas, so be aware that ticks are present. Ticks, which are arthropods and not insects, need a host to feast on in order to reproduce. The ticks that light onto you while hiking will be very small, sometimes so tiny that you won't be able to spot them. Primarily of two varieties, deer ticks and dog ticks, they need a few hours of actual attachment before they can transmit any disease they may harbor. Ticks may settle in shoes, socks, or hats and may take several hours to actually latch on. The best strategy is to visually check every so often while hiking; do a thorough check before you get in the car; and then, when you take a posthike shower, do an even more thorough check of your entire body. Ticks that haven't attached are easily removed but not easily killed. If you pick off a tick while on the trail, just toss it aside. If you find one on your body at home, remove it and then send it down the toilet. For ticks that have embedded, removal with tweezers is best.

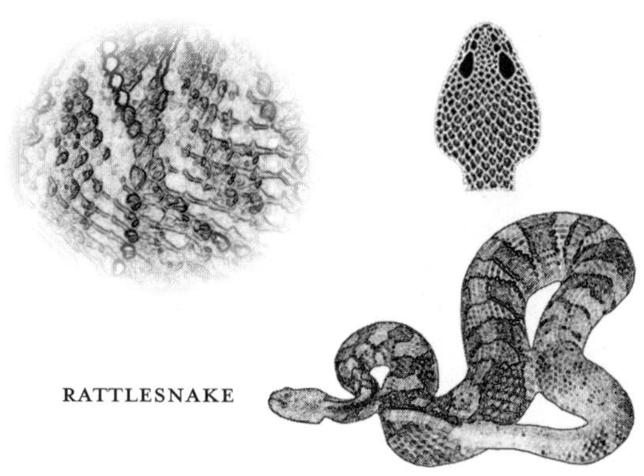
RATTLESNAKE

Snakes

Four types of rattlesnakes inhabit Anza-Borrego Desert State Park. Always be on the lookout for snakes; if you see one, give it plenty of room and leave it alone. When snakes have the opportunity, they escape from sight before you are upon them. Because snakes sense vibrations, a hiking stick pounded along the ground as you walk gives them fair warning of your presence and allows them to slither off. This tactic is probably why I have never seen a rattler in the park—a fact that amazes almost everyone I tell. Countless others have shared their stories of encounters with rattlers in the desert, so I know they're plentiful. But the only snake I've seen is the coachwhip, a non-venomous snake that nonetheless can give a nasty bite if provoked.

When hiking in rocky areas, be careful where you step or put your hands. Fallen leaves also provide a hiding place, so be careful as you walk through them. As with any wild animals, snakes are drawn to available water, so you may be more likely to encounter them near streams.

Mountain Lions

In some areas of the park, you will see signs indicating that mountain lions (also known as cougars) are present. In my desert treks, I've seen lots of tracks, so I am always alert for the predators. Encounters with mountain lions are rare, but whenever you venture into an animal's habitat, the possibility exists. If you do see a mountain lion, leave it alone. More than likely, it will want to get out of sight. Here are a few helpful guidelines for mountain lion encounters:

- Keep your children close to you, or hold your child. Observed in captivity, mountain lions seem especially drawn to small children.
- Do not run from a mountain lion. Running may stimulate the animal's instinct to chase.
- Do not approach a mountain lion. Instead, give him room to get away.
- Try to make yourself look larger by raising your arms and/or opening your jacket if you're wearing one.
- Do not crouch or kneel down. These movements could make you look smaller and more like the lion's prey.
- Try to convince the lion you are dangerous—not its prey. Without bending or crouching down, gather nearby stones or branches and toss them at the animal. Slowly wave your arms above your head and speak in a firm voice.
- If all fails and you are attacked, fight back. Hikers have successfully fought off an attacking lion with rocks and sticks. Try to remain facing the animal, and fend off attempts to bite at your head or neck—a lion's typical aim.

Poison Oak

Although uncommon, poison oak does exist in the desert. The only hike included in this book where I've encountered this nasty plant is in Oriflamme Canyon (see page 105). But conditions do change. Where water is present, you may find poison oak—recognized by its three-leaflet configuration—on either a vine or shrub. Urushiol, the oil in the sap of this plant, is responsible for the rash. Usually within 12 to 14 hours of exposure (but sometimes much later), raised lines and/or blisters will appear, accompanied by a terrible itch. Refrain from scratching, because bacteria under fingernails can cause infection

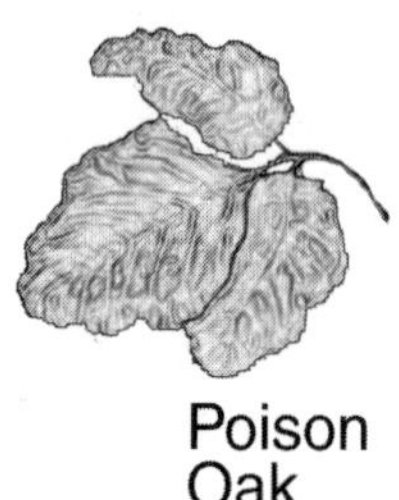

and you will spread the rash to other parts of your body. Wash and dry the rash thoroughly, applying a calamine lotion or other product to help dry the rash. If itching or blistering is severe, seek medical attention. Remember that oil-contaminated clothes, pets, or hiking gear can easily cause an irritating rash on you or someone else, so be sure to wash not only any exposed parts of your body but also any exposed clothes, gear, or pets.

Tips for Enjoying Anza-Borrego Desert State Park

I've chosen to include some of the best and most popular areas in Anza-Borrego Desert State Park, giving you an overview, then narrowing those regions to my favorite hikes. Within each write-up, you'll find descriptions of area plants and perhaps a quirky detail or two about how they grow or how Native Americans used them. You'll read information about specific birds and other animals, as well as a little bit of history if such information applies. I've also included some geological specifics and landmarks such as nearby mountains, historical sites, or the source of water you'll find on the trail.

To get specific information before you go, visit **www.parks.ca.gov** or **www.anzaborrego.statepark.org,** or call the park at (760) 767-5311. Dropping by the Visitor Center, with its well-stocked bookstore, and getting guidance from rangers will also be time well spent, because knowledge and preparation can keep you safe—and being safe allows you to have fun. Here are a few more tips for enjoying your time in the desert.

• **TAKE YOUR TIME ALONG THE TRAILS.** Anza-Borrego Desert State Park is filled with wonders both big and small. Don't rush past a bright-pink flower to get to that overlook. Stop and examine the beautiful swirled striations in a nearby rock, or notice the patterns etched into the sand by tiny footsteps. Let the sound of a rushing stream trickle joy into your mood, and don't be so focused on getting to the hike's end that you miss its middle. Short hikes allow you to stop and linger more than long ones—something about staring at the front end of a 10-mile trek naturally pushes you to speed up. That said, take close notice of the elevation maps that accompany each hike. If you see many ups and downs over large altitude changes, you'll obviously need more time. Inevitably, you'll finish some of the hikes long before or after the suggested times. Nevertheless, leave yourself plenty of time for those moments when you simply feel like stopping and taking it all in. Some of my most memorable conversations have been during impromptu stops with a friend along the trail.

• **WE CAN'T ALWAYS SCHEDULE OUR FREE TIME** when we want, but try to hike during the week and avoid the traditional holidays if possible. Trails that are packed in the spring, when wildflowers are at their height, are often clear during the colder months. Though the flowers aren't as plentiful, you'll almost always find some in bloom. If you are hiking on a busy day, go early in the morning; it'll enhance your chances of seeing wildlife.

Backcountry Advice

Please practice low-impact camping. Adhere to the adages "pack it in, pack it out," and "take only pictures, leave only footprints." Practice "leave no trace" camping ethics while in the park.

Solid human waste must be buried in a hole at least 3 inches deep and at least 200 feet away from trails and water sources; a trowel is basic backpacking equipment.

These suggestions are intended to enhance your experience within the confines of this state park. Regulations can change over time; contact the park to confirm the status of any regulations before you enter the backcountry.

Trail Etiquette

Whether you're on a city, county, state, or national park trail, always remember that great care and resources (from nature as well as from your tax dollars) have gone into creating these trails. Treat the trail, wildlife, and fellow hikers with respect.

- HIKE ON OPEN TRAILS ONLY. Respect trail and road closures (ask if not sure), avoid possibly trespassing on private land, obtain permits and authorization as required, and leave gates as you found them or as marked.
- LEAVE ONLY FOOTPRINTS. Pack out what you pack in. No one likes to see the trash someone else has left behind.
- NEVER SPOOK ANIMALS. An unannounced approach, a sudden movement, or a loud noise startles most animals. A surprised animal can be dangerous to you, to others, and to the animal itself.
- PLAN AHEAD. Know your equipment, your ability, and the area in which you are hiking—and prepare accordingly. Be self-sufficient at all times; carry necessary supplies for changes in weather or other conditions.
- BE COURTEOUS TO OTHER HIKERS, bikers, equestrians, and all those you encounter on the trails.

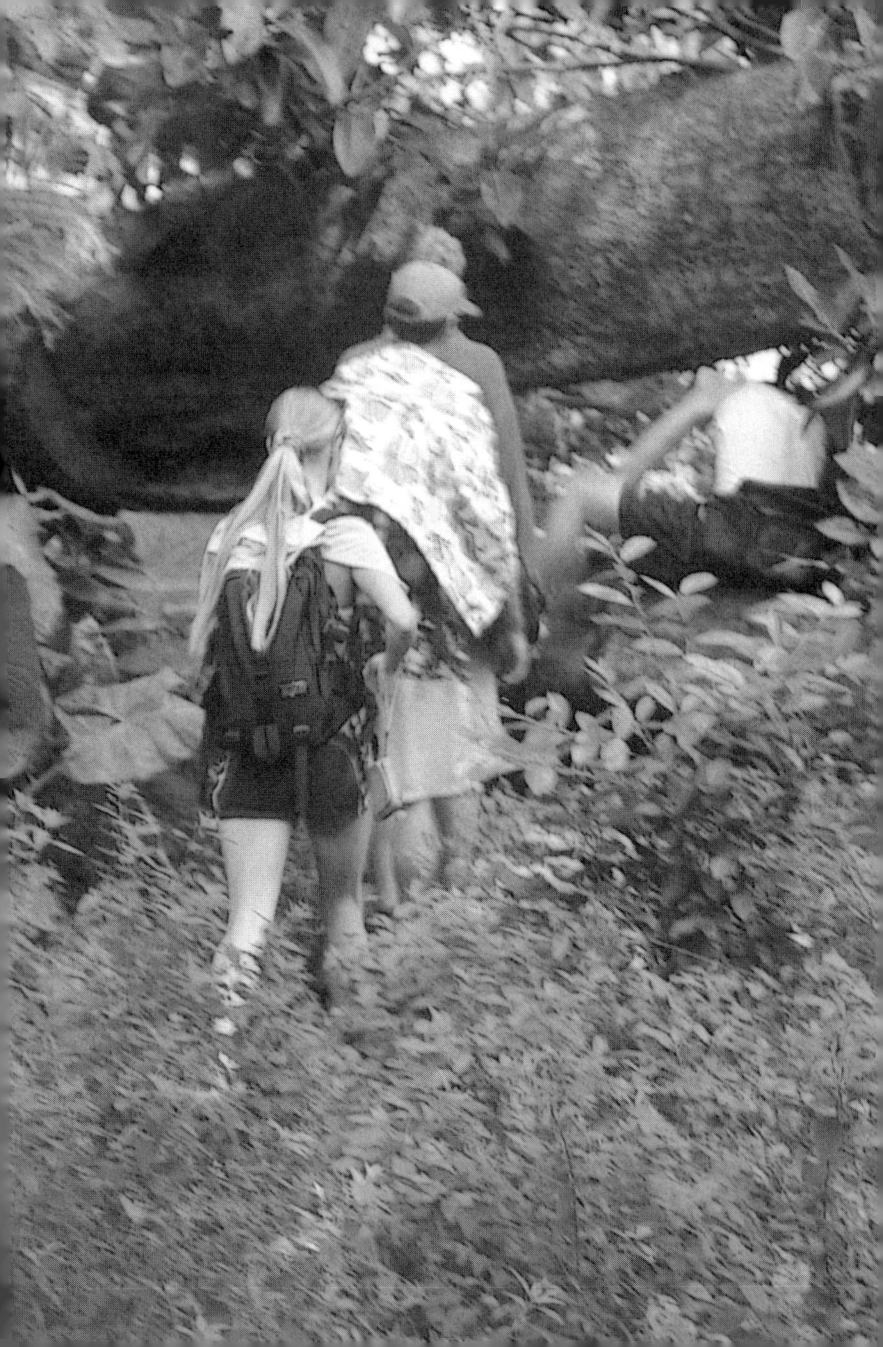

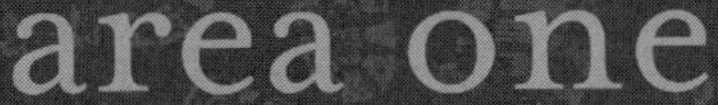

area one

CULP VALLEY, HELLHOLE CANYON, AND BORREGO PALM CANYON

Many consider the desert dry and desolate but secret oases cool waterfalls interesting animals and a wide array of adaptive vegetation wait quietly to refresh adventurous souls

AREA 1: CULP VALLEY, HELLHOLE CANYON, AND BORREGO PALM CANYON

Introduction

CULP VALLEY, HELLHOLE CANYON AND PALM CANYON are all accessible from County Route S22, more commonly known as Montezuma Valley Road. Some of the easiest hiking and camping to get to within Anza-Borrego Desert State Park, these areas are also some of the most popular. Expect fellow nature lovers in mild-weather months and crowds on weekends during the spring blooming season.

A number of springs in Culp Valley make for fertile areas that contrast with the surrounding boulders and arid landscape. A wonderful big-sky atmosphere permeates the region, allowing for views of drifting clouds that shadow the Borrego Valley down below. At an elevation of more than 3,000 feet, Culp Valley sometimes sees snow when the temperatures dip. Winter hiking is especially entertaining for this reason.

Culp Valley Primitive Camp is north of Montezuma Valley Road, but you'll find people tent camping almost anywhere in the area. Pulloffs along dirt Jeep routes not far from the highway make the area popular for convenient overnight and weekend stays.

Hikes included from the Culp Valley area include trails to Pena Spring, a leg of the California Riding and Hiking Trail, and the Wilson Trail. You could also hike or four-wheel-drive the Jasper Trail and hoof it into Tubb Canyon (both south of Montezuma Valley Road), with an eye for overnight tent camping.

A few miles further down steep Montezuma Valley Road, you'll find Hellhole Canyon on your left. A large turnout with restrooms provides access to the 0.5-mile Surprise Canyon Loop (a favorite for Sunday drivers looking for spring blooms and not interested in much exercise or energy expenditure), the trek to refreshing Maidenhair Falls, and a strenuous climb suitable only for experienced hikers to an oasis in Flat Cat Canyon. A trail from Hellhole Canyon also leads a mile or so northwest to the Visitor Center.

Borrego Palm Canyon, with its well-developed campground (117 individual sites, 52 for RVs), nature trail, and close proximity to the Visitor Center, is the most visited canyon in Anza-Borrego Desert State Park. Despite my long forays into very remote areas filled with sheep tracks, here on this nature trail with lots of people around is where I've seen the endangered bighorns. Sightings are fairly common along the stream.

The nature trail leads to a large oasis where most people turn and head back. If you're an experienced, physically fit hiker, you'll enjoy a deeper trek into Borrego Palm Canyon, perhaps to camp. With its remarkable displays of striated rock, plentiful oases, and rushing water, Borrego Palm Canyon is one of the most beautiful places on Earth.

1 Wilson Trail

SCENERY: ✩✩	DISTANCE: *8.7 miles round trip*
DIFFICULTY: ✩✩✩	HIKING TIME: *4–5 hours*
TRAIL CONDITION: ✩✩✩✩	OUTSTANDING FEATURES: *Predominantly flat with some hills and dales, wildflowers in spring, horned lizards, rock formations, view of the desert valley and the Salton Sea*
SOLITUDE: ✩✩✩✩✩	
CHILDREN: ✩✩✩	

Because access to the trailhead is off Old Culp Valley Road, which requires a four-wheel drive past the first 0.25 miles, the Wilson Trail offers plenty of solitude and peaceful communion with nature. You will probably see lots of overnight visitors during mild-weather months camping along Old Culp Valley Road. Once on the trail, though, your footsteps echo off surrounding brush in the otherwise-still silence of this long, fairly easy trek. (There are a few very short semisteep sections.) The three-star difficulty rating is for length.

OPTION: *You could pack in supplies and camp overnight near the peak. Fall asleep with stars twinkling overhead and the yip-yip serenade of coyotes. Hike the 5.5-mile return trip in the morning. Or turn around at the viewpoint and return the same day.*

From the trailhead, move southeast on a narrow footpath that descends a little, levels out, then gradually climbs, setting the pattern for most of this steady south-southeast hike. After a short distance, two narrow, rutted tracks split by vegetation show that this is an old Jeep route. The path is named for early Ranchita cattle rancher Alfred Wilson.

During my last visit, fresh mountain-lion tracks made their way along the first 2 miles of trail. Large boulder clusters would perhaps make good hiding places for the cats, so be aware of your surroundings. In Anza-Borrego Desert State Park, you're in their habitat.

Wilson Trail

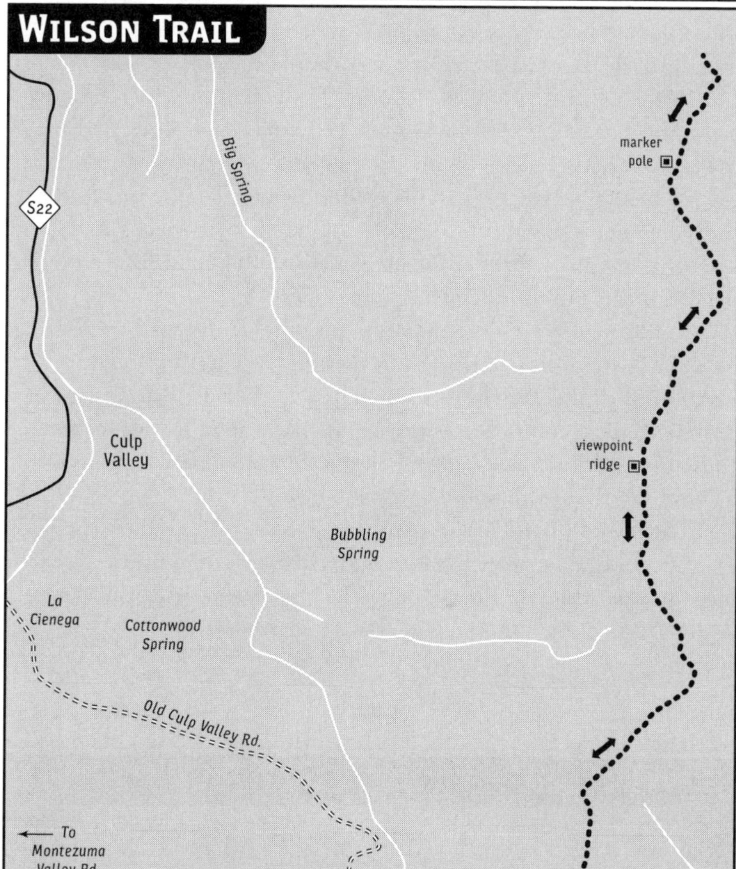

S22

Big Spring

marker pole

Culp Valley

viewpoint ridge

Bubbling Spring

La Cienega

Cottonwood Spring

Old Culp Valley Rd.

To Montezuma Valley Rd.

S22

To CR S22 and Ranchita

N

0 4000

Feet

The first 3.5 miles require easy, gradual climbing interspersed with dips and level spots. A couple of short stretches climb slightly more quickly, but you can power over those with general ease.

In springtime, you may encounter bee swarms, perhaps hearing only their buzzing. Or you may duck as the swarm abruptly darkens the air around you. Despite the bad rap bees sometimes get, swarming is a benign activity. When the colony grows too large for the hive, the queen departs and is followed by others who will form a new hive in a new place. Bees pollinate plants and flowers, filling a much-needed niche and thus deserving our respect.

A short, steep section at around 3.8 miles climbs past interesting boulder formations to a ridge with views of the Culp Valley and surrounding hills. Watch for horned lizards. The docile reptiles are prevalent, their coloration matching the rocky sand for protection. Indian legend links one's grandfather to horned-lizard sightings, so be kind. Your ancestors may be watching you!

The trail dips and levels, continuing for another mile through easy terrain lined with yellow blooms in spring. You'll begin to see more juniper trees on the cholla-packed land and perhaps discover coyote tracks along the trail (the scat is everywhere).

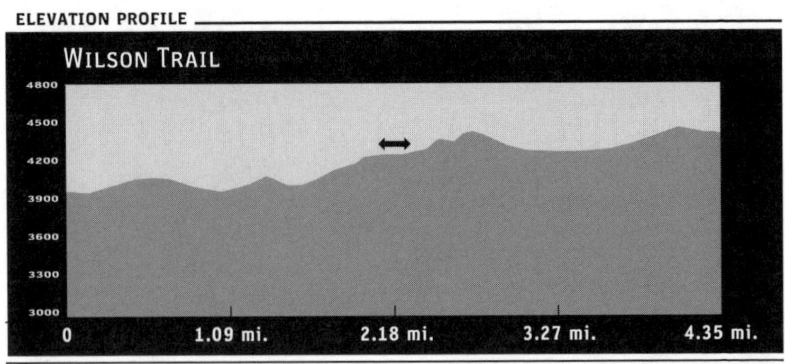

At 5 miles, you will come to a wooden pole. Set in a clump of concrete loosened from the soil, the pole is usually lying on the ground. Visitors prop it up with heavy, bowling ball–sized rocks, but wind and weather inevitably knock the marker flat again.

The trail narrows, climbing 0.25 miles to the right up a rocky path lined with fragrant piñon pine, juniper, manzanita, and jojoba before it levels. The 4,573-foot Wilson Peak will be on your right, looking less than formidable at the trail's already high elevation of around 4,500 feet. You will have climbed close to 700 feet from the trailhead, a hardly noticeable distance as it is spread over more than 5 miles.

The path levels into a plateau and continues east for another quarter mile or so, then evaporates as the land begins to dip. Head left to boulder outcroppings just a few yards north of the trail, and glimpse Borrego Springs in the distant valley. To the northeast, the Salton Sea, California's largest lake, stretches out like a misty blue ribbon.

This is a good place to catnap on the rocks or pause for lunch. If you've packed in overnight supplies, set up camp. Then sit back and relax as the shadows lengthen and eclipse the light, giving way to velvety twilight and the bright sparks of the stars and moon.

Directions: From County Route S2, turn left on S22 (Montezuma Valley Road, also known as Montezuma Highway) and drive 10 miles east to Old Culp Valley Road. Turn right onto this dirt road that quickly becomes rutted and hilly. Switch to four-by-four mode and follow the main route (ignoring offshoots to the right or left) for about 2.6 miles. A small turnaround loop circles a lone juniper on the left, where you'll spot the sign marked "Wilson Trail." (Go too far and you'll come to a sign marked "The Slab," which is 0.1 mile past the trailhead.)

GPS Coordinates	1 WILSON TRAIL
UTM Zone (WGS84)	11S
Easting	548103
Northing	3672898
Latitude–Longitude	N 33° 11' 37.9151"
	W 116° 29' 2.1647"

2 Hellhole Canyon to Maidenhair Falls

SCENERY: ☆☆☆☆
DIFFICULTY: ☆☆☆
TRAIL CONDITION: ☆☆☆
SOLITUDE: ☆☆☆
CHILDREN: ☆☆☆☆

DISTANCE: *5.2 miles round trip*
HIKING TIME: *4.5 hours*
OUTSTANDING FEATURES: *Sandy wash, ocotillo, cholla cactus, agave, seasonal stream, and waterfall with maidenhair ferns*

At first glance, this may seem just another dry, flat hike, but the desert holds surprises. Spend the last mile or so hopping on boulders to find a shady palm oasis with a waterfall lined in cascading maidenhair ferns.

From the trailhead staging area, move generally southwest toward the mountains, starting on a flat wash of sandy soil through desert chaparral. At around 0.3 miles, reach a split in the trail. Take the right-hand route (the left begins an arduous climb to the Culp Valley Overlook on the California Riding and Hiking Trail; see page 38). Several yards past this split, you may also notice an ill-defined trail heading north—this leads to the Anza-Borrego Desert State Park Visitor Center, about a mile away.

As you march along, take note of the sounds around you—not much but the *crunch-crunch-crunch* of your footsteps in the porous desert ground. In the early morning, you might be lucky enough to see a jackrabbit or two darting behind a greasewood bush. Seeing these rabbits is exciting for visiting hikers, but to the Indians living in the area years ago, the rabbits were garden pests. The ocotillo you'll notice reaching heavenward with its spine- and leaf-lined arms was a useful native plant. By cutting off the long limbs, lining them up around gardens, and watering them, the Native Americans encouraged branches to take root, providing an effective living fence against the hungry jackrabbits that damaged their gardens.

At about 0.5 miles, the trail bears slightly to the right, quickly moving back to its generally southwestern route. The mountain rises

HELLHOLE CANYON TO MAIDENHAIR FALLS

To Palm Canyon Drive

CR&H Trail junction

Visitor Center trail junction

Montezuma Valley Rd.

S22

Flat Cat Canyon turnoff

Hellhole Canyon

Hellhole Palms Trail

Flat Cat Canyon Trail

Flat Cat Canyon

Hellhole Palms

first palms

Maidenhair Falls

N

0 2400

Feet

on the right, blocking some sunshine and ensuring that Hellhole Canyon remains cooler in the morning hours.

Teddy bear cholla becomes more prevalent, groups piling almost on top of one another to appear like spiny villages. In the afternoon, sunlight glistens over the numerous spines, making the cacti look fuzzy, like a teddy bear.

After approximately 1.25 miles, bigger boulders begin to dot the trail, foreshadowing a mile-long section of rock hopping required to reach the falls. At first, the boulders only encroach the trail in spots, providing steps up and down as you progress.

As you move up the canyon, look for topographical evidence of floodwaters on the terrain. The trail comes close to the water-etched washout to the right. A sign warns that this is mountain-lion territory. Be aware of your surroundings, as the possibility of an encounter always exists. A recent visit revealed fresh tracks along the sand wash, but no animal sightings.

You are, however, likely to tangle with catclaws of the plant variety. The wiry stems of this small tree, a member of the acacia family, have feathery leaves and sharp "claws" that grab at clothing and skin.

At a little more than a mile, the trail veers north, with a flat area

ELEVATION PROFILE

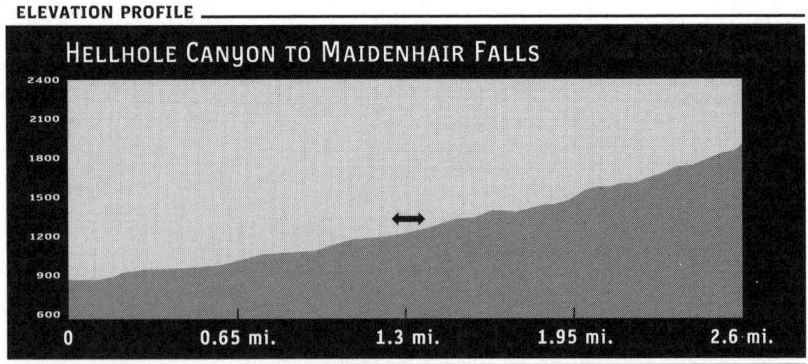

appearing to continue that direction. If you wanted to hike into adjacent (and extreme) Flat Cat Canyon, you would go that way. Instead, take the narrower trail leading to the left (southwest).

Past the 1.5-mile mark, the trail crosses the channeled-out sand wash, then crosses back again. Watch for the tubular red flowers of the chuparosa, which grow on a gray-green mound-shaped bush. Conserving energy in the arid climate, chuparosa lack leaves during much of the year, but the bright flowers often bloom profusely after rains. The Spanish word *chupar* means "to suck," which is what hummingbirds do to the nectar-filled flowers.

With their food source, nectar, present in abundance, hummingbirds are plentiful. In the dense quiet of a desert-canyon hike, listen for the call of the purple-crowned Costa's hummer. The male's drawn-out, high-pitched vocalization is surprising, sounding like the whine of a dentist's drill.

The boulders become bigger and more plentiful and as the well-defined trail ends, some rock hopping begins. A sycamore tree appears, and you'll spot a few palms ahead in the ravine alongside more sycamores.

The first palm grove is a good place to turn around if you're averse to boulder hopping. Weigh the effort against what's ahead—only 0.5 miles remain to reach the falls, which are a delight. As you hike around boulders and up over those that require some climbing, flat sections of trail reappear for short stretches. Pass through areas where water trickles, making its way down the canyon. In the late fall, the sycamore leaves turn a tangerine orange, lighting up the drab, rocky landscape.

When you reach Maidenhair Falls, you'll recognize it for its namesake. Even when drier weather prevents a heavy pour of water from the approximately 18-foot drop, lacy green ferns cascade down the rock face in abundance. The area surrounding the falls is like a private, shaded garden where few rays of sunlight penetrate the canopy of palm fronds and sycamore leaves. Grapevines grow in a wooded tangle up through the trees, their fleshy leaves hanging in bunches like yellow-green leis. In fact, if led here blindfolded, upon seeing the site you might be momentarily tricked into believing you'd reached a tropical paradise.

Maidenhair Falls is a favorite on hot days after rains when water flows heavily, but a gentle trickle is more relaxing. In the chilly shade of this desert oasis, sit and listen to the constant song of myriad droplets. Even the smaller amounts of water, flowing steadily beneath the exposed rock, pleasantly rumbles like the distant echo of thunder.

Before heading back the way you came, pause and etch the beauty of this natural sanctuary into your mind. This way, on stressful days back in civilization, you can call up the calming image for relaxation.

Directions: From Interstate 15, take the Pala–Highway 76 Exit and drive east for 33.6 miles to CA 79. Turn left, traveling 4.1 miles to County Route S2, where you'll turn right and drive another 4.6 miles to CR S22–Montezuma Valley Road (commonly called the Montezuma Highway). Turn left. Drive approximately 14 miles to the trailhead on the left, which sits almost 1 mile south of the Visitor Center.

GPS Coordinates	2 HELLHOLE CANYON TO MAIDENHAIR FALLS
UTM Zone (WGS84)	11S
Easting	555319
Northing	3678938
Latitude–Longitude	N 33° 14' 52.8130" W 116° 24' 22.1743"

3 Flat Cat Canyon

SCENERY: ★★★	DISTANCE: *5 miles round trip*
DIFFICULTY: ★★★★★	HIKING TIME: *6–7 hours*
TRAIL CONDITION: ★	OUTSTANDING FEATURES: *Desert flowers, rock formations, expansive view of the desert valley, palm oasis, and trickling water*
SOLITUDE: ★★★★★	
CHILDREN: NOT RECOMMENDED	

This extreme trek up a densely vegetated, boulder-populated ravine offers a sense of accomplishment at hike's end. But expect a tough climb, eking out a route as you scale boulders toward a hidden palm oasis at 2,500 feet (a 1,700-foot elevation gain). Don't attempt this hike unless you're experienced and physically prepared for a tough challenge; also, make sure you have plenty of water and lots of time for a slow, grueling pace. Ravine temperatures can drop significantly from those on the desert floor, so wear layers to escape a chill. Also consider a double layer of pants to protect your skin from tangles with prevalent and unforgiving acacia catclaw. And be aware of any expected bad weather—you don't want to get caught in this steep canyon ravine in storms and flooding.

From the trailhead staging area, move generally southwest toward the mountains on the Hellhole Canyon Trail (see Hellhole Canyon to Maidenhair Falls, page 28). After 1.2 miles, head north on the flat path, away from Hellhole Canyon. Move toward the narrower, adjacent (to the north) canyon; this is Flat Cat Canyon, named for a dead "flat" bobcat found by rangers in a cavern near the top many years ago.

At first, this less-defined route may make you feel as if you're cutting aimlessly across open desert. Don't worry—you haven't fallen down Alice's rabbit hole, though you may glimpse the long ears of a jackrabbit loping among the cholla cacti and the silver-green mounds of chuparosa. Also watch for small, shallow depressions in the sand. These are the dusty "tubs" made by kangaroo rats that roll in the sand to bathe.

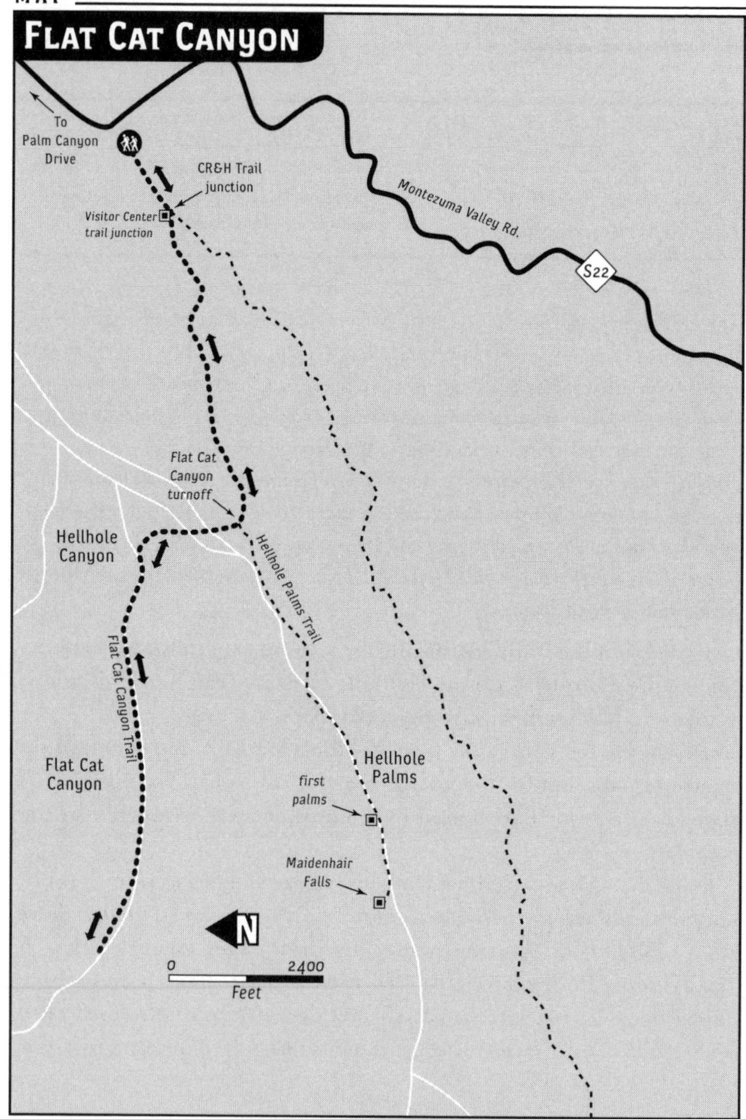
Flat Cat Canyon
To
Palm Canyon
Drive
CR&H Trail
junction
Visitor Center
trail junction
Montezuma Valley Rd.
S22
Flat Cat
Canyon
turnoff
Hellhole
Canyon
Hellhole Palms Trail
Flat Cat Canyon Trail
Flat Cat
Canyon
Hellhole
Palms
first
palms
Maidenhair
Falls
N
0
2400
Feet

Cut across a sand wash channeled out by floodwaters, and turn to the right for a short distance. Tracks are usually plentiful in this area. You're likely to see the hoof prints of bighorn sheep, along with coyote and fox tracks, which are difficult to tell apart. A coyote's claws are usually more defined on imprint than a fox's.

The (southern) ridge of Flat Cat Canyon will be on your left. At its rocky endpoint, take a look at the interesting metamorphic rock that looks like enormously magnified phyllo dough, its many layers baked a deep brown. Head north again for a short distance, then southwest into the ravine's opening. The trail will be what you make of it at first, picking your way through cacti and rocks.

Generally, the best way to start heading up the ravine is on the right, where a gently ascending sand wash makes for fairly easy stepping (heading more to the left requires more-difficult rock scrambling).

Watch for birds' nests in the spindly trees and bushes (acacia, palo verde, creosote). The verdin, a small, yellow-capped bird native to the desert, builds a globed nest with an opening near the bottom. On outer tree limbs you may see a few nests in close succession; the male verdin builds several of them so his mate can choose the one in which they'll raise their young.

Also look for spring flowers, sometimes blooming even in fall and winter after rains. Dark-purple desert Canterbury bells bear yellow stamens. Bright desert gold poppies rise from fringelike leaves. Magenta-pink monkey flowers with darker magenta markings and gold-yellow stamens provide low-growing splashes of color.

A few stands of boulders that you can step over give way to less readily scaled ones. As the hike progresses, you'll be required to puzzle out the best handholds and steps to ascend the canyon. Among increasing boulder problems and nasty tangles of catclaw bushes, the route is slow going. You'll see the leavings of canyon-dwelling wood rats near rock crevices. The piled deposits of elongated oval droppings are called "middens," although the creatures themselves remain unseen.

A nice little ledge about 1.75 miles from the trailhead is a good place to pause and gaze down at your progress thus far. The desert valley is distant, the cars moving along Montezuma Valley Road almost soundless from this vantage point. Perhaps stop to rest and have a drink or snack. You'll hear and see hummingbirds. Ravens fly overhead, and you might spot quail. With binoculars, take in close-up views of the rocky ridges on either side of the canyon. You might get lucky and spot a group of well-camouflaged bighorns resting on a rocky ledge.

The next 0.25 miles or so is difficult terrain. Moving to the left side of the gorge is a little easier going at this point—*easy* being a relative term on this challenging hike. Once you scale a couple of difficult boulder sets, you'll come to a flat, open area. The terrain lasts only about 60 yards, so savor the moment. Be sure to look up into the ravine. This is your first opportunity to spot the palm oasis peeping into view. Tired and sweaty, you may have begun to doubt its existence. Spotting those palm fronds peeking above a boulder may feel like finding buried treasure, or how Columbus must have felt upon finally spotting land. Even for the most experienced, this extreme hike is a challenging adventure.

Only a little more than 0.5 miles remain to reach the palms, but don't get too confident (and possibly careless). Quite a few demanding

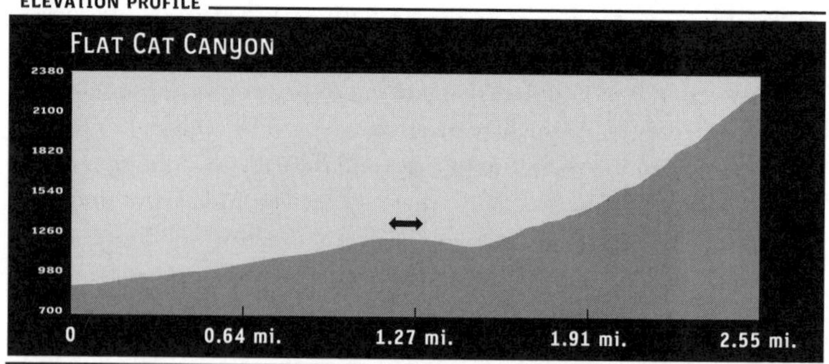

boulder puzzles remain. Moving steadily, you'll need 40 minutes or more to reach the first palm tree.

Staying left remains the easier route. Past the first palm, work your way down into the center of the narrow canyon. From there, you'll reach several more palms, where water trickles around and over rocks. Be careful, watching every step. A pile of jumbled rocks forms a cavernlike space here. Before realizing it, you may find yourself stepping over its top. Fallen palm fronds don't provide solid footing, and spaces between the rocks could easily allow a foot to slip through, causing injury.

You can continue a little farther to the largest grove of palms if you're up to more exertion, or finish the hike in the shade near any one of the smaller groupings. A vee of light-revealing sky above the desert valley is your view from the dim shade of the oasis.

The canyon towhee (a grayish-brown bird with reddish underside highlights) may hop close, curious to have a look at the new visitors. The perky bird's wings taunt you as it flits away. Contemplating the trip down, you may wish you could sprout a set of wings yourself—for an easy descent. Be sure to give yourself plenty of time (two and a half to three more hours) for the return trip.

Directions: From Interstate 15, take the Pala–Highway 76 Exit and drive east for 33.6 miles to CA 79. Turn left, traveling 4.1 miles to County Route S2, where you'll turn right and drive another 4.6 miles to CR S22–Montezuma Valley Road (commonly called the Montezuma Highway). Turn left. Drive approximately 14 miles to the trailhead on the left, which sits almost 1 mile above the Visitor Center.

GPS Coordinates	3 FLAT CAT CANYON
UTM Zone (WGS84)	11S
Easting	555319
Northing	367893
Latitude–Longitude	N 33° 14' 52.8130"
	W 116° 24' 22.1743"

4 California Riding and Hiking Trail

SCENERY: ☆☆☆
DIFFICULTY: ☆☆☆☆
TRAIL CONDITION: ☆☆☆
SOLITUDE: ☆☆☆☆
DISTANCE: *7.4 miles round trip*
HIKING TIME: *7–8 hours*
OUTSTANDING FEATURES: *Steady ascent and descent with spring wildflowers, desert vegetation, breathtaking views of the desert valley, and wildlife*

Springtime wildflowers, interesting year-round cacti and boulder formations, plentiful wildlife, and an isolated atmosphere make this strenuous hike a paradise for those in good physical condition. A steady climb up (and then down) the sandy, rocky trail can make this walk grueling. Windy weather can be dangerous on the narrow, sometimes-steep trail.

OPTION: *For a shorter one-way hike, you could take two cars in a shuttle, parking one at the top at the Pena Springs pullout and leaving the other at the trailhead down below.*

From the trailhead staging area, move generally southwest toward the mountains, starting on a flat wash of sandy soil through desert chaparral spotted with cholla cactus. Ocotillo is also present, reaching heavenward with its spiny arms bedecked with lipstick-red blooms. Less than a mile in, you'll come to a split in the trail. Head left (the right-hand route will take you to Maidenhair Falls), and the trail narrows, beginning its zigzagging ascent.

Steadily climb through boulder outcroppings baked brown by the desert sun and heat. In the early mornings, and later on cold winter days, the fog-filled valleys open in the distance, giving an otherworldly feel to the hike.

As the trail's elevation rises, the ocotillo plants thin, leaving hedgehog and cholla cacti as surrounding mainstays. Some cactus varieties are short and stout; others are taller and lined in protective spines the size of toothpicks (be careful). With your mind free of citified clutter, let your imagination go, finding animals and other

California Riding and Hiking Trail

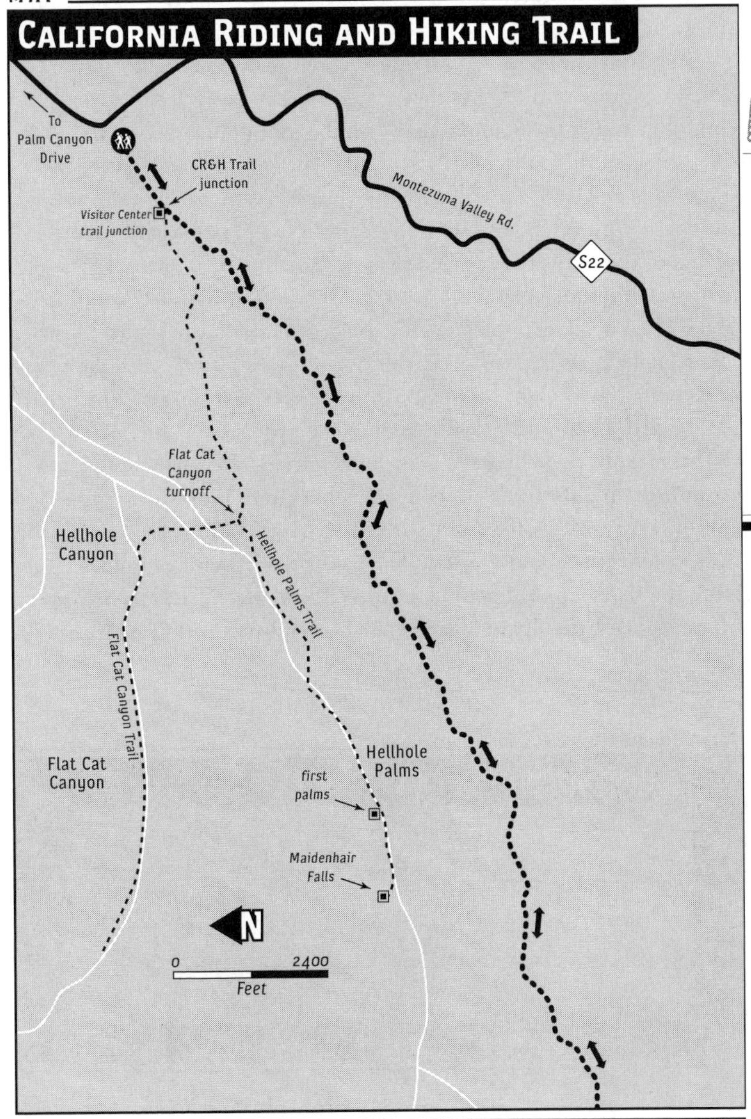

shapes within the cacti and rock formations—nature likes to have fun, and so should you!

Around 3 miles up, you'll descend a little on the rocky trail, continue uphill awhile, then reach a flat wash area—welcome after climbing. Watch for bighorn sheep on the mountainsides. Well camouflaged, they aren't easily spotted. You're more likely to see their tracks near the trail, which prove the elusive creatures share this desolate space. You might also see bobcat tracks (or perhaps get a glimpse of one of them, more likely in the early morning or evening). Low-flying quail skitter by in large groups. On a recent visit, a coachwhip snake raced by. The quick-moving snake was little more than a blur but identifiable by its dark color and the way it carries itself—with the front of its body raised high, on the lookout for prey as it hurries along.

Continue climbing. Wide steps of flat ground and trail offer restful meanderings between gains in elevation. Towering boulder groupings on either side of the route all begin to look alike as you continue upward. Don't search for trail markers, which become virtually nonexistent past about 2 miles. The trail isn't difficult to follow from the valley up, but people heading downward near Pena Springs often report difficulty in locating the descending route. Roadrunners

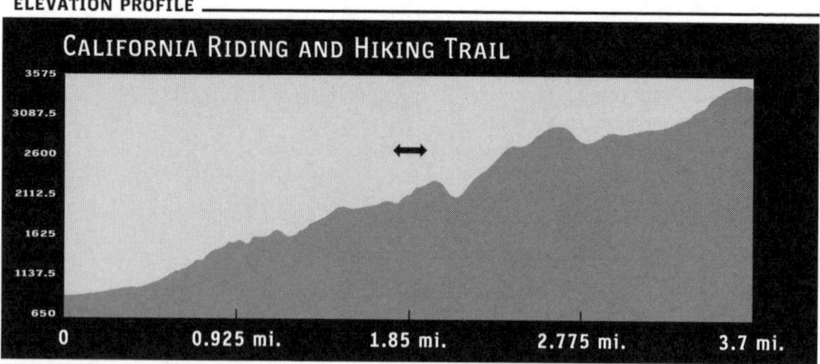

hop among the rocks, their long tail feathers flicking up and down, balance ballasts for their quick movement up the rocks.

The short viewpoint trail to the Culp Valley Overlook comes as a surprise when you finally reach it. It's marked by a sign on the left and a yellow-topped California Riding and Hiking Trail pole. The view is spectacular, but after the long journey through a desolate landscape, the overlook can be anticlimactic. The Pena Springs pullout trail, which leads just 0.5 miles from Montezuma Valley Road to the overlook, is often busy, prompting hikers who've spent the last three or four hours in quiet, nature-nurtured thought to head back down the mountain and its solitude. Be sure to enjoy views of the valley as you descend.

The hike up might have logically seemed the more difficult trek, but your body may tell you otherwise at the end of the day. Descending on the sometimes steep, narrow trail lined with cacti means putting on the brakes and, in gusty desert winds, requires attention to every step. Your lower legs, tendons, and toes may backtalk later. Once you're at home, a hot soak and a fluffy pillow pave the way to a good night's sleep—dreaming of your next visit to Anza-Borrego Desert State Park.

Directions: From Interstate 15, take the Pala–Highway 76 exit and drive east for 33.6 miles to CA 79. Turn left, traveling 4.1 miles to County Route S2, where you'll turn right and drive another 4.6 miles to CR22–Montezuma Valley Road (commonly called the Montezuma Highway). Turn left. Drive approximately 14 miles to the trailhead on the left, which sits almost 1 mile above the Visitor Center.

GPS Coordinates	4 CALIFORNIA RIDING AND HIKING TRAIL
UTM Zone (WGS84)	11S
Easting	555319
Northing	3678938
Latitude–Longitude	N 33° 14' 52.8130" W 116° 24' 22.1743"

5 Borrego Palm Canyon Nature Trail

SCENERY: ☆☆☆
DIFFICULTY: ☆
TRAIL CONDITION: ☆☆☆☆
SOLITUDE: ☆
CHILDREN: ☆☆☆☆☆

DISTANCE: *3 miles round trip*
HIKING TIME: *2–2.5 hours*
OUTSTANDING FEATURES: *Desert-wash landscape, stream and waterfalls, birds, possible bighorn-sheep sightings, and a shady oasis*

Use the interpretive guide found at the trailhead to identify plants, animals, and other desert phenomena along this easy, well-visited desert-wash nature trail.

Grab a trail guide at the kiosk adjacent to the restrooms, and head northwest on this short loop into desert wonder. You'll begin in typical wash landscape—sand and small boulders alongside a large "wash" basin where water may or may not be flowing. The trail is relatively flat, with a few short steps up or down over bowling ball–sized boulders (some a bit larger or smaller), heading through cholla-studded land. If the stream is running, you'll cross it for the first time at around 0.33 miles before continuing northwest.

As you walk along this easy trail, listen for birdcalls. You may see quail running in groups, their wings like an explosion of applause if they take off en masse. Notice also the deep-brown color on the rocks forming the canyon walls. This "desert varnish" is the result of bacterial colonies that fasten themselves to the rocks. The brown stain was thousands of years in the making. Keep watch also for the elusive Peninsular bighorn sheep. The endangered animals' brown coats blend in with the varnished rocks, making them difficult to see. But they are present and often spotted along this busy nature trail—sometimes dashing right across the path in front of you (as has happened to me).

At approximately 0.66 miles, watch for a marker sign leading you to the left, up to higher ground and then down again, closer to the stream that runs in winter and spring. At around 0.8 miles, the

Borrego Palm Canyon Nature Trail

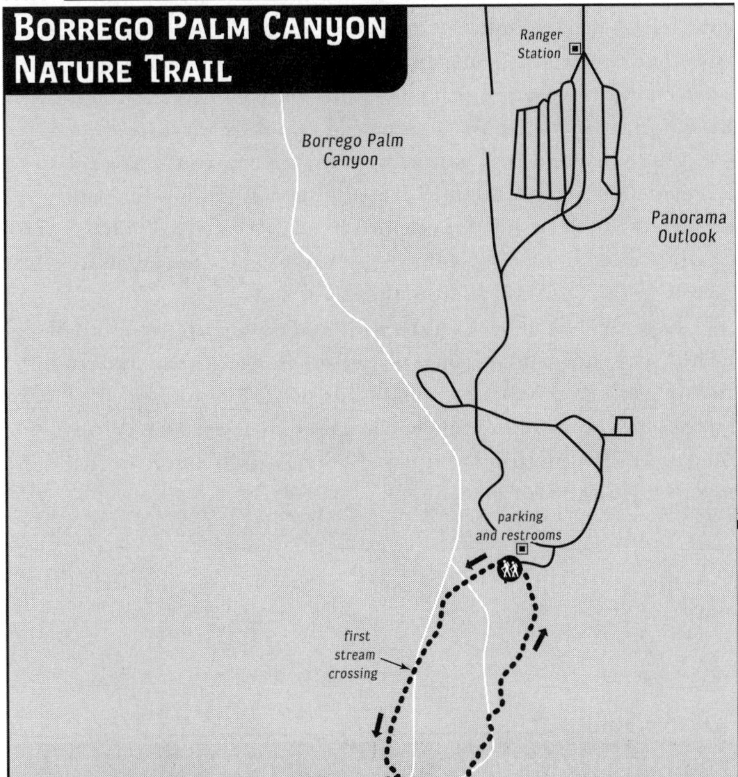

Ranger Station

Borrego Palm Canyon

Panorama Outlook

parking and restrooms

first stream crossing

cross to west side of stream

oasis and end of Nature Trail

To Visitor Center

N

0 2400

Feet

route crosses to the west side of the stream. Once across, look to your left. A marker indicates an alternate trail. This leg was added later than the original nature trail, making for a loop or balloon-on-string configuration that allows another route back to the trail-head. Ignore this for now, turning right on the path instead.

On the narrow trail to the left of the stream, you'll pass a few large boulder groups, some with cascading falls. Follow the path clear to the oasis, a wide area shaded by a large cluster of fan palms. Spend as long as you like at the oasis. You're likely to see lots of other people in this cool refuge from the desert sun.

To return, head back on the path to the alternate trail, following its hill-and-dale pattern generally southwest back to the trailhead. Before leaving, examine the man-made pupfish pond near the kiosk and read about this Pliocene-epoch species that was here before the desert. The pupfish has survived because of its ability to adapt to a changing environment.

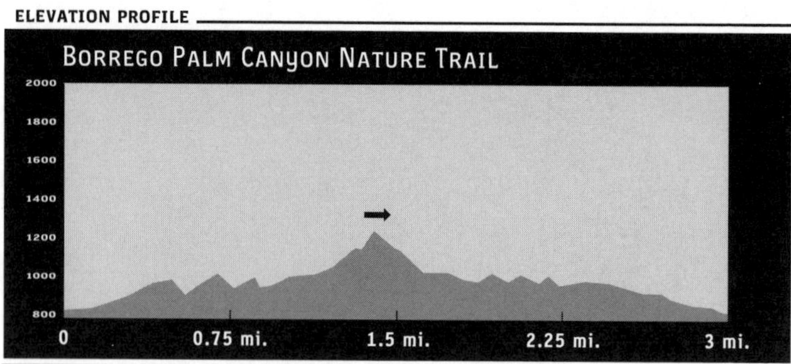

Directions: From Interstate 15, take the Pala–Highway 76 exit and drive east for 33.6 miles to CA 79. Turn left, traveling 4.1 miles to County Route S2, where you'll turn right and drive another 4.6 miles to CR S22–Montezuma Valley Road (also known as the Montezuma Highway). Follow S22 to Palm Canyon Drive, and turn left. Then take the first right (almost immediately), following this paved access road approximately 1 mile to the campground entrance. Pay for day use at the Ranger Station on your way in; then drive (veering right) to the end of the road. Parking is adjacent to the restrooms, which are at the trailhead.

GPS Coordinates	5 BORREGO PALM CANYON NATURE TRAIL
UTM Zone (WGS84)	11S
Easting	554181
Northing	3681407
Latitude–Longitude	N 33° 16' 13.1900" W 116° 25' 5.6166"

6 Borrego Palm Canyon to South Fork Falls

SCENERY: ☆☆☆☆☆	DISTANCE: *9 miles round trip*
DIFFICULTY: ☆☆☆☆	HIKING TIME: *6–6.5 hours*
TRAIL CONDITION: ☆☆	OUTSTANDING FEATURES: *Huge, beautiful slabs of colorful schist and gneiss rocks (some of which you'll climb on and over), running stream, palm oases, and waterfalls*
SOLITUDE: ☆☆☆☆	
CHILDREN: NOT RECOMMENDED	

Don't let the easy terrain of the Borrego Palm Canyon Nature Trail, where you begin this rugged hike, fool you: it's not for beginners. The Nature Trail's benign, well-trodden path, which ends at the first oasis, doesn't begin to hint at the sometimes-daunting, always-beautiful solitude of a deeper venture into the canyon. Wear long pants and sleeves to protect against acacia catclaw bushes. Layered clothing to stay comfortable is always a good idea when trekking into remote areas where rock walls sometimes block sunlight and warmth. Grip-soled, waterproof hiking boots can also be useful, since a single misstep during one of several stream crossings can mean several miles in soggy shoes. If you're day-hiking, plan extra time to enjoy the serenity of this craggy, awe-inspiring terrain.

OPTION: *Backpacking in for an overnight stay is fairly common, and you'll spot others' campsites in wider canyon sections, particularly where palms and sycamores grow. Awakening to the babble of water running over stones, the call of crows, and the soft rustle of palm fronds fits into a nature lover's dreamscape.*

Start out on the Nature Trail as described in the previous hike. When you reach the first palm grove, though, pass through the oasis and venture beyond the "end of trail" sign. You can do this by scrambling over the big, pale boulders just beyond the oasis, or take a small side trail to the left, climbing onto the ridge and then back down through thick desert willows and past the huge rocks beyond the palms. Either way, you'll find a fairly decent route (I won't call this an actual trail, but foot tracks lead the way) on the south side of the stream.

MAP

Borrego Palm Canyon to South Fork Falls

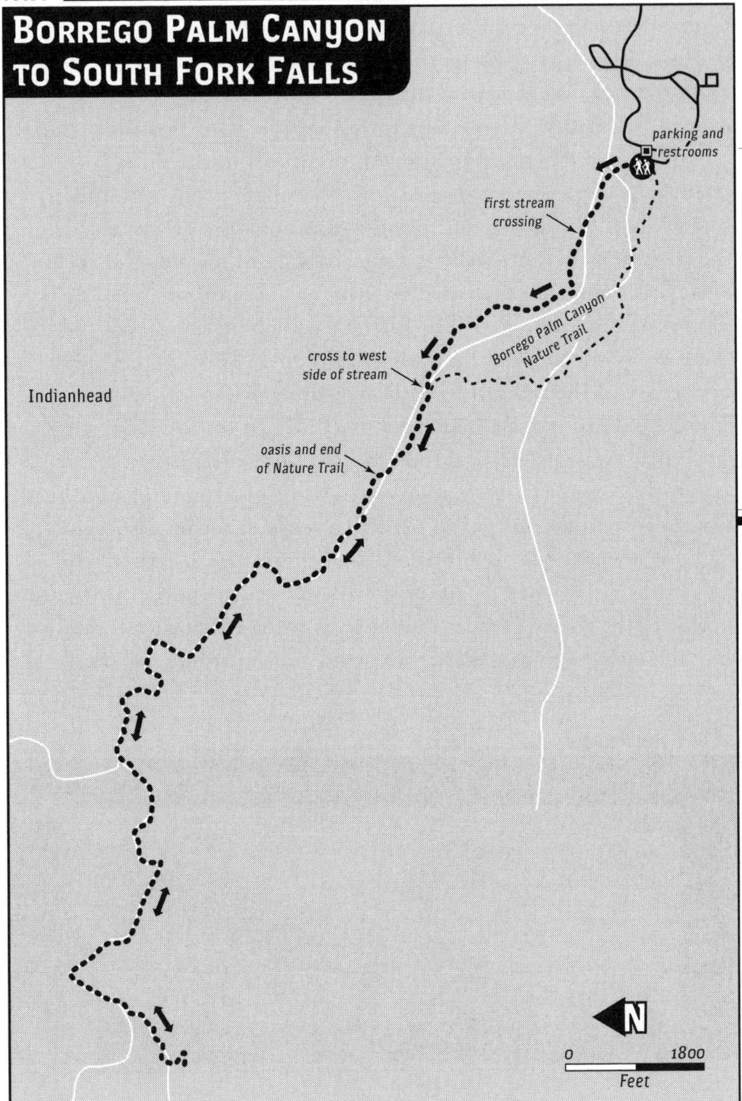

parking and restrooms

first stream crossing

Borrego Palm Canyon Nature Trail

cross to west side of stream

Indianhead

oasis and end of Nature Trail

N

0 1800
Feet

Near the first bend in the canyon, more large boulders await. Carefully climb over these, perhaps getting your feet wet in the process. As you progress up the canyon, you'll need to cross back and forth over the stream as the land requires, usually with ease, on smaller, flattish stones. Again, you may get your feet wet at times.

The second bend in the canyon occurs around 2 miles from the trailhead, where the surrounding rock will have taken on rainbow hues. You'll be picking your way through boulders on either side of the stream, sometimes walking on giant slabs of the colorful rock. Near this point, huge, slanted slabs narrow in around a rushing fall. To traverse this area, you'll be forced to climb up several feet, where there are numerous flat footholds in the rock. Some hikers walk briskly across the footholds, seemingly oblivious to any danger. Those afraid of heights (like me!) will find this section harrowing. The safest strategy is sitting and scooting on the slanting surface, aware of the water rushing across hard stone eight to ten feet below. Once you get past this point, revel in a sense of accomplishment, and put the challenge behind you—that is, until your return trip!

Enjoy the bright strip of sky above rocky canyon walls, the chanting babble of the rushing water, and the interesting rock patterns reminiscent of swirls, rainbows, and zebra print. Watch for bighorn sheep.

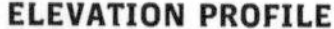

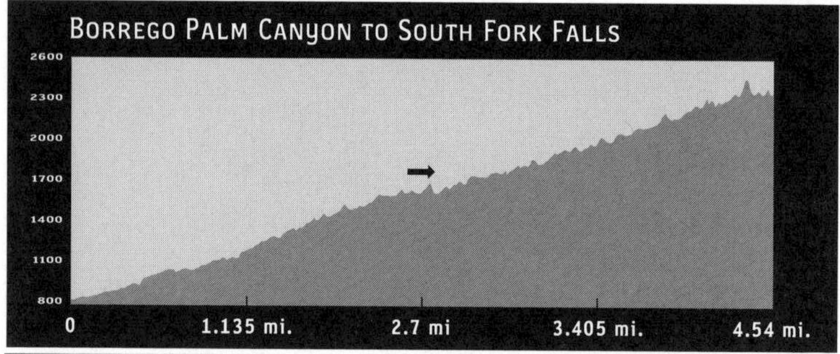

At around 2.5 miles, a smaller ravine comes in from the north. Pass this by, continuing west. Palm groves dot the canyon as you follow the stream, passing through sections where water pools in tree shade, gurgles over smaller rocks, and rushes around larger boulders.

At around 3 miles, you'll begin to see sycamore trees and palms. In the fall, their gold-orange leaves add a splash of color. The stream forks at around 3.4 miles. Take the South Fork stream on the left, which moves southwest (Palm Canyon continues northwest). Here, reeds and willows grow in thick, lush stands. Standing pools are covered in duckweed, making you forget you're in the desert. You may have to forge your own path through the greenery, hopping the stream where necessary, but remaining mostly on its north (right) side for approximately another 0.33 miles. Be careful not to disturb this plant and wildlife habitat any more than necessary; also, note that the exact types of vegetation you'll see depend on what has regrown after the canyon was scoured out by a postfire flood in 2004. Smaller falls partially hidden by the overgrowth splash over boulders, leading to the turnaround point—falls of approximately 30 feet.

When you're ready to return, retrace your steps, forever influenced by memorable Borrego Palm Canyon.

Directions: From Interstate 15, take the Pala–76 exit and drive east 33.6 miles to CA 79. Turn left, traveling 4.1 miles to County Route S2, where you'll turn right and drive another 4.6 miles to CR S22–Montezuma Valley Road (also known as the Montezuma Highway). Follow S22 to Palm Canyon Drive, and turn left. Then take the first right (almost immediately), following this paved access road about 1 mile to the campground entrance. Pay for day use at the Ranger Station on your way in; then drive (veering right) to the end of the road. Parking is adjacent to the restrooms, which are at the trailhead.

GPS Coordinates	6 BORREGO PALM CANYON TO SOUTH FORK FALLS
UTM Zone (WGS84)	11S
Easting	554181
Northing	3681407
Latitude–Longitude	N 33° 16' 13.1900"
	W 116° 25' 5.6166"

area two

COYOTE CANYON

Many
consider
the
desert
dry
and desolate
but
secret oases
cool
waterfalls
interesting
animals
and
a wide
array of
adaptive
vegetation
wait
quietly
to refresh
adventurous
souls

Introduction

Coyote Canyon is a huge cleft that runs along the San Jacinto earthquake fault between the San Ysidro and Santa Rosa mountains and hosts perennial Coyote Creek. The constant creek flow starts in Riverside County's Santa Rosa Wilderness, south of 8,716-foot Toro Peak. The waterway's long downhill stretch flows through Coyote Canyon, ending in Borrego Sink, which at less than 500 feet is the lowest point in the Borrego Valley.

Coyote Canyon's copious amounts of water attract wildlife and feed abundant flora and fauna in this isolated, yet favorite, recreational playground. Because of the continuous presence of water, recreational use of Coyote Canyon is controlled to safeguard wildlife. Seasonal closure June 1 through September affords the endangered Peninsular bighorn sheep and other wildlife a dependable and undisturbed water source.

Located in the northwest corner of Anza-Borrego Desert State Park, the fertile region was once home to the so-called coyote people, a sect of the Cahuilla Indians. Beginning in the late 1700s, California colonists began traveling through the area, an obvious natural passage through the mountains. During the next hundred years or so, the presence of outsiders, resulting skirmishes, and the introduction of smallpox eventually drove these Native Americans from the area.

Today, thousands of Californians and out-of-state visitors come to Coyote Canyon to enjoy horseback riding, camping, hiking, and four-wheeling. Although the dirt road running through the canyon used to serve as a thoroughfare, a central 3-mile stretch between Middle Willows and Upper Willows is now closed to vehicles year-round to protect sensitive habitat. (It remains open to foot traffic.)

Other areas within the canyon are also permanently closed to vehicle traffic, preserving the wild character of Coyote Canyon and its fertile grottoes filled with trickling waterfalls.

For clarity, let me tell you how to get to Coyote Canyon and prepare you for your day and overnight experiences in this stunning region. All but two of the trails included here are accessed via the directions below. Horse Canyon and White Wash are accessed from the more remote park entrance near the town of Anza in Riverside County. For more specific directions, see the individual write-ups for Horse Canyon and White Wash (pages 74 and 78), which include a brief overview of additional hiking and camping opportunities in that area.

To get to Coyote Canyon from the quaint town of Borrego Springs, drive east on Palm Canyon Drive (approximately 2.5 miles from the Visitor Center, or 0.5 miles from Christmas Circle) to paved DiGiorgio Road, and turn left. After approximately 5 miles, DiGiorgio Road's pavement ends. From this point, civilization all but vanishes. You'll quickly cross a sometimes-muddy wash area, and continue northwest with Coyote Mountain to your right. At 2.5 miles from the pavement's end, you'll notice Alcoholic Pass, a hiking trail not included in detail here, but worth a look if you have the time and inclination. The rocky trail gains around 600 feet over the first mile and offers views northeast to the Santa Rosa Mountains and southwest to the San Ysidro Mountains. You may be wondering about the name, which historians say may have derived from the trail's use as a shortcut into Borrego Springs for drinks. Just over 0.5 miles farther on the dusty sand road brings visitors to Desert Gardens, a popular picnic spot, on the right.

At approximately 3.5 miles, the unpaved road comes to the first crossing of Coyote Creek. The stream is usually running here, and although many vehicles have little trouble fording the creek at this initial crossing, some drivers choose to park in the ample turnout space. Depending on the condition of the road and the crossing, which can change due to weather, continued road travel may be iffy.

On weekends in the busy late-winter and early-spring desert recreation season, you'll likely begin seeing tent campers from this point forward. The open camping policy in all of the park (except close to streams) makes Coyote Canyon a hot spot for quick getaways, not only for those who want to hike to the canyon's more remote areas, but for people who choose a more just-off-the-road experience. Sheep Canyon Primitive Campground, only mildly more civilized than open camping in a spot of your choice, is another option—about 4 miles past the third crossing (6 miles from the first).

Just under 5 miles from the pavement's end, the second crossing appears. If you're not in a four-wheel-drive vehicle, consider stopping here. Less than a mile forward, you'll see a large parking area on your left, just prior to the third crossing. Even those in four-wheel drives often stop here, choosing to hoof it across the stream into the Lower Willows area and beyond. The road itself veers abruptly left and intersects the stream, but even if you make it through this third crossing with the most water flow, what lies ahead may give you pause. The road moves over a steep section, paved by nature with large and jutting boulders. Many an oil pan leaves its greasy mark on these boulders, and you'll routinely see four-wheel drives turning back at the base of the steep, rocky hill. It's fun to stand and watch the ones that try, adding yours to the hoots and hollers of those who make it—and your sympathy to those who don't!

The detailed write-ups I've included from the Coyote Canyon area range from an easy, looping stroll through marshy Lower Willows to more rugged hikes holding treasures well worth the extra effort, such as Sheep, Cougar, and Indian canyons. If you're in a four-wheel drive and can make it past the third crossing, you can drive 4 miles to a vehicle closure point that offers quicker, easier access to these watery canyons.

In the remote northwestern corner of the park, I've outlined trips leading into Horse Canyon and into White Wash. If you're after solitude, try the sampling I've included here. But be prepared—the road going down into the park is nothing less than horrendous, even for four-wheel drives. Warning signs remind visitors that tow trucks and emergency vehicles won't go down the rocky road. Even the hardiest gung-ho off-roaders won't likely consider the hairpin turns over slippery rocks on steep overhangs a fun experience. A turnout a short distance from the park's entry gate may be the rest-easy ticket—except that you'll be walking down, then back up, the steep Anza trail.

7 Lower Willows Loop

SCENERY: ☆☆☆
DIFFICULTY: ☆☆
TRAIL CONDITION: ☆☆
SOLITUDE: ☆☆
CHILDREN: ☆☆☆☆

DISTANCE: *4.2 miles round trip*
HIKING TIME: *2 hours*
OUTSTANDING FEATURES: *Running water; people on horses; soft, sandy trail alternating with dry, dusty path; and dense willow thickets*

The loop through the willows in this marshy area lures people by the thousands each season. Don't come here looking for solitude, although you may find such serenity on a weekday or for a few moments within a dense willow patch that blocks the sound and presence of others. The trail on this easy hike alternates between muddy, sandy, and dust-kicking to the point of covering your nose and mouth with a bandana. The route's qualities depend on weather and water flow, traveling through cool, shaded willow thickets, then out onto the Jeep road and past a historical marker. Typical desert oases make one think of palm trees, but this is an oasis of a different sort. The ever-present water and wooded landscape provide refuge to animals such as the red-spotted toad and such rare birds as the least Bell's vireo.

Leave your vehicle in the parking turnout on the left, just prior to the third crossing (see the Coyote Canyon Introduction, page 52). Walk northwest a short distance, and when you see the sign marking the third crossing, head across to the left. You can either ford the stream in its open part, where the vehicles do, or take one of the narrow, tunnel-like paths snaking through the willows. Once across, you'll see the sign marking the entrance to Lower Willows. Turn right onto the dusty trail. This is the official trail opening and the logical way to go, but it's also the busiest. For more solitude, take a less definable route (that leads to the same place) by continuing northwest from the third crossing sign. Instead of fording the stream, make a path of your own (very little of Anza-Borrego is off limits to

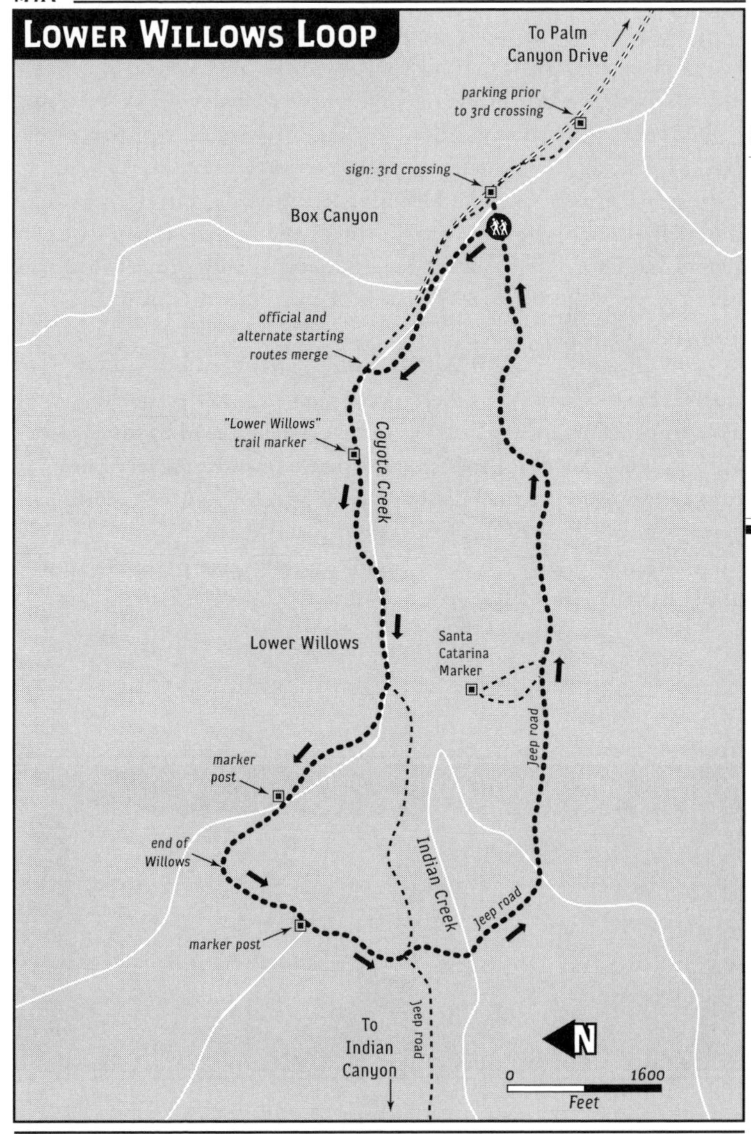
Lower Willows Loop
To Palm Canyon Drive
parking prior to 3rd crossing
sign: 3rd crossing
Box Canyon
official and alternate starting routes merge
"Lower Willows" trail marker
Coyote Creek
Lower Willows
Santa Catarina Marker
Jeep road
marker post
end of Willows
Indian Creek
Jeep road
marker post
Jeep road
To Indian Canyon
N
0
1600
Feet

those on foot), or follow meandering footsteps northwest for about 800 yards, where you can hook up with the official trail anyway. Both routes meet, then cross the creek and continue in the shade of dense willows rising like brushy walls on either side of the cool, shaded trail.

At approximately 0.5 miles, the path reaches a marker that reads "Lower Willows," then bends on a more westerly route. Continue, moving out of shade now and likely encountering a dusty portion of trail that will have you covering your nose and mouth. If you have a bandana, here's your cue to use it. Sunglasses help protect your eyes in the loose, well-churned silt that flies up and forms dust clouds with every step.

On my visits to Lower Willows, wildlife has been evident yet elusive. Early-morning or dusk hours offer the most promising opportunity for spotting animals in this area well trod by humans, but you'll hear birds calling from the dense cover of the trees any time of day. And the tracks of bighorn sheep, coyotes, and raccoons mark their presence in this water-rich area.

At approximately 1.6 miles, you'll find a marker post at the end of the strip of willows that crowd around Coyote Creek. Turn left

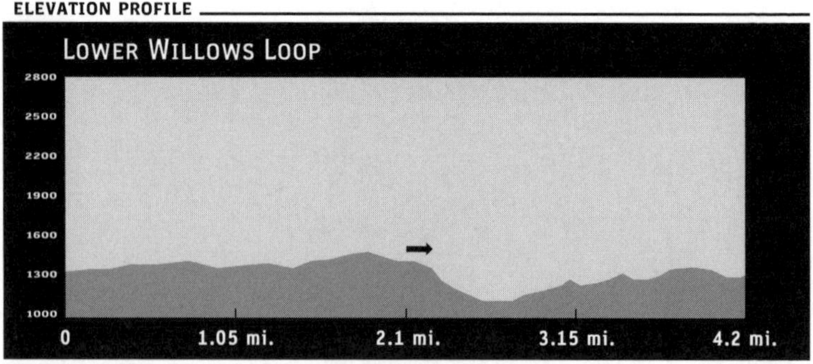

here. The path moves southwest, connecting to another marker post less than 0.25 miles away. You'll reach an open area and a line of posts on your right that closes off the protected Lower Willows area to vehicles. Cross the wide, sandy space and follow the pole arrows pointing southwest. The trail climbs a small bluff, connecting to the Jeep road at just over 2 miles. At the road, turn left and head east alongside the vehicle route, while enjoying long views of open desert filled with yellow-blooming creosote with its tiny fuzz-ball fruits.

Approximately 0.8 miles after turning onto the Jeep road, an 0.1-mile side trail leads to a historical marker offering information about Santa Catarina Spring, named by Juan Bautista. This explorer led the first overland route from Mexico to California, and his group camped by the spring during their journey. From the bluff where the monument sits, you can look out and search for the spring, but all that's clearly visible is the dense strip of willows you encountered up close on the Lower Willows trail.

From the side trail, the Jeep road climbs some. Near its crest, be sure to look back to the west for a stretching view of Coyote Canyon framed by distant mountains. The vast space formed by this fault-line gap is breathtaking.

Directions: From Borrego Springs, drive east on Palm Canyon Drive and turn left on DiGiorgio Road. Drive 5 miles till the pavement ends; then continue on the dirt road for an additional 5.6 miles to the large turnout on the left, just before the third crossing. If you cannot or choose not to drive all the way to this point, park at the first or second crossing, adding appropriate mileage to the hike (see the Coyote Canyon Introduction, page 52).

GPS Coordinates	7 LOWER WILLOWS LOOP
UTM Zone (WGS84)	11S
Easting	553631
Northing	3692616
Latitude–Longitude	N 33° 22' 17.24" W 116° 25' 24.48"

8 Sheep Canyon

SCENERY: ★★★★★	DISTANCE: *2–10 miles round trip*
DIFFICULTY: ★★★★	HIKING TIME: *4–7 hours*
TRAIL CONDITION: ★★	OUTSTANDING FEATURES: *Variety of waterfalls, massive and unusually shaped boulders, oases, and lush riparian environment*
SOLITUDE: ★★★★	
CHILDREN: ★	

A daylong out-and-back hike from the third crossing parking area, or 2 round-trip miles if your four-wheel drive can make it to Sheep Canyon Primitive Camp. Whichever you choose, Sheep Canyon is a rugged trek holding picturesque settings at every turn. Abundant water cascades from massive boulder formations and shady caverns.

OPTIONS: *Flat, sandy spots in the canyon's wide areas make good campsites that don't break the park's rules about camping too close to water sources. Or make use of Sheep Canyon Primitive Camp, and then access the trailhead in the early-morning hours, when wildlife is most active.*

From the parking area just before the third crossing (see the Coyote Canyon Introduction, page 52), turn left and cross the stream, pass by the entrance to Lower Willows, and continue up the steep, rocky hill heading west. The rocky uphill section continues for about 0.66 miles before the road begins a gradual descent. On foot or by four-wheel drive, continue west on the Jeep road. It's about 1.5 miles till you pass the spur road on the right leading to the Santa Catarina Spring historical marker. The road bends a little to the right. Continue along this dirt Jeep route, as directed by the "Sheep Canyon" marker sign. At just more than 2 miles, the road forks; follow the left split west toward a sign marked "Sheep Canyon Camp." At approximately 3.8 miles from the third crossing, the route dips, crossing a wide, sandy wash. Turn right at the turnoff to Sheep Canyon Primitive Camp at 4 miles. There's plenty of space

Sheep Canyon

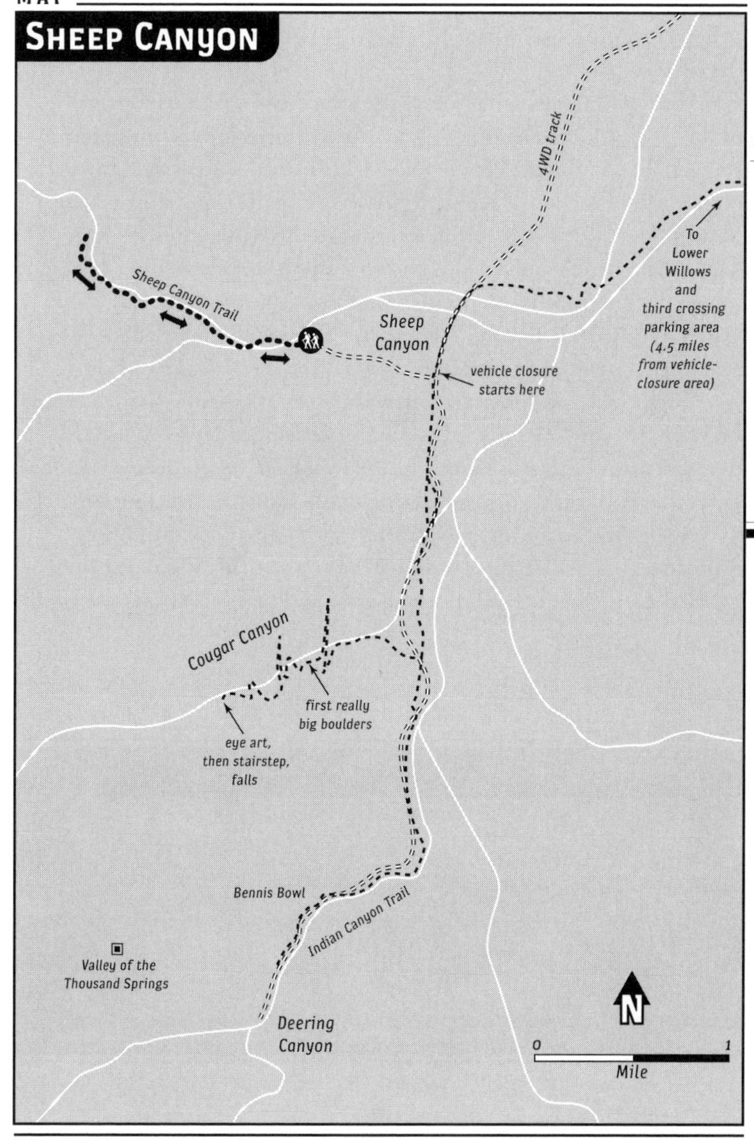

Sheep Canyon Trail
Sheep Canyon
4WD track
vehicle closure starts here
To Lower Willows and third crossing parking area (4.5 miles from vehicle-closure area)
Cougar Canyon
first really big boulders
eye art, then stairstep, falls
Bennis Bowl
Indian Canyon Trail
Valley of the Thousand Springs
Deering Canyon
N
0
1
Mile

to park here, or you can drive a short distance to the end of the official camping site, where you'll see the hiking trail. We'll call this the official trailhead.

Head past the metal horse tie into the canyon via a narrow path to the right, which takes you to sand dunes running between stream fingers. The trail moves toward the right (north) side of the canyon, crossing the stream or keeping it just to the right (depending on the water's flow). Generally, if you stay toward the right, you'll be fine. The stream bends to the right, and you'll note a canyon fork coming in on the right—which is where you want to go. The south fork of Sheep Canyon is straight ahead, but going there is not recommended—it's easy to get caught in inescapable "bowls" formed by massive rocks.

Turn right and generally follow the stream, crossing so the water is on your left now. You'll need to climb over embedded boulders that pave the path (fairly easy, with some handholds). Sycamores and willows encroach, with gentle breezes adding to the sound of trickling water.

At 0.2 miles, an idyllic waterfall comes into view, tumbling around a huge rectangular boulder that's an anchoring point for a gnarled cottonwood, several sycamores, and palms. Pass on the right,

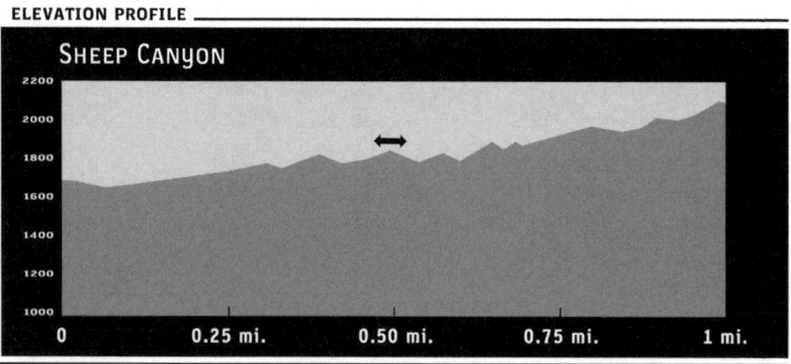

climbing over boulders and using trees for handholds. Or squeeze by on the left, without as much vegetation to hang on to.

Look for the signs of ant-lion larvae in small sandbars gathered atop and alongside the boulders. The tiny, cone-shaped pits are the voracious ant lion's way of trapping the smaller insects on which they feed. As adults, the larvae form cocoons from which they later emerge as lacy-winged flying insects.

You'll pass beneath oak trees, reveling in their dense shade as well as that of sycamores and palms. The rock canyon wall rises on your left, with the fleshy, succulent chalk live-forever clinging like pale-green bows. Cross the stream as many times as you need to, noticing baby cottonwoods by the hundreds. Climb encroaching boulders as necessary, careful where and how you step—snakes could be resting in the fallen leaves. Also be aware that what looks like solid ground may not always be: piled rocks covered in leaf litter can hold hollows. One misstep recently sent my foot—*whoosh*—down an unseen hole. In an instant, my leg had disappeared into a cavern formed by piled boulders.

At about 0.33 miles, a large waterfall cascades over steplike rocks. From here, you'll need to cross and recross the stream as it meanders down the canyon. Just follow the lay of the gorge, which reaches a 25- to 30-foot waterfall at 0.4 miles. The water flows from some large angled boulders, arranged to form a wet cavern below. Pass this boulder-crowded area by climbing a little on the right side of the canyon, angling back toward the steam, then crisscrossing back and forth over the sparkling water—perhaps with tree frogs hopping.

About 0.5 miles from the trailhead, boulders again encroach, making it necessary to go right, then arc back toward the stream. Here, the mother of all boulders, shaped like the great stern of a ship, comes into view. A huge, gnarled sycamore blocks passage on the right, so to go any farther, you'll have to climb up around the boulder on the left. This is difficult, but worth it. Just a few yards past the ship boulder is a large, cool cavern, its ceiling formed by another massive boulder. Enjoy the shade and the echoes of water tumbling in, around, and through piled rock. Sunlight reaching through crevices causes a dancing reflection on the stone ceiling in this cool, dripping space.

From the large cavern, the canyon comes to a fairly quick end. Heading to the left, you can scramble carefully up the rocks to a saddle for a perched view down the canyon if you choose. In warmer weather, leaving behind the watery caverns and shady oaks in favor of a sweaty rock climb won't often appeal. Retrace your steps back down the valley, careful as always to avoid a fall—and to enjoy the delightful sights and songs of nature.

Directions: From Borrego Springs, drive east on Palm Canyon Drive and turn left on DiGiorgio Road. Drive 5 miles till the pavement ends; then continue on the dirt road for an additional 5.6 miles to the large turnout on the left, just before the third crossing. If you cannot or choose not to drive all the way to this point, park at the first or second crossing, adding appropriate mileage to the hike (see the Coyote Canyon Introduction, page 52). In a four-wheel drive, it's possible to begin the hike 4 miles from the third crossing at the Sheep Canyon Primitive Camp—cutting this hike by 8 miles round trip.

GPS Coordinates	8 SHEEP CANYON
UTM Zone (WGS84)	11S
Easting	548157
Northing	3691995
Latitude–Longitude	N 33° 21' 57.9924"
	W 116° 28' 56.4475"

9 Cougar Canyon

SCENERY: ☆☆☆☆☆	DISTANCE: *3.5–11 miles round trip*
DIFFICULTY: ☆☆☆☆	HIKING TIME: *4.5–7 hours*
TRAIL CONDITION: ☆☆	OUTSTANDING FEATURES: *Variety of waterfalls, huge boulders, wildlife, oases, and rock art*
SOLITUDE: ☆☆☆☆	
CHILDREN: NOT RECOMMENDED	

A daylong hike from the parking area at the third crossing, or a shorter foray if your four-wheel-drive vehicle can make it to the vehicle closure just past Sheep Canyon Primitive Camp. Whichever you choose, Cougar Canyon is a watery treasure trove. Waterfalls are the norm here, with a new variation in size and flow at every turn on this uphill trek into a fertile gorge.

OPTIONS: *Plenty of flat, sandy spots in the wider portions of the canyon make good campsites that don't break the park's rules about camping too close to water sources. If you do spend the night, you'll be serenaded by the sound of falling water magnified by the lack of ambient noise. Pick a place that sounds pleasant to you. In some spots, abundant water is almost deafening.*

From the parking area just before the third crossing (see the Coyote Canyon Introduction, page 52), turn left and cross the stream, pass the entrance to Lower Willows, and continue up the steep, rocky hill heading west. The rocky uphill section continues for about 0.66 miles before the road begins a gradual descent. On foot or by four-wheel drive, continue west on the Jeep road. It's about 1.5 miles till you pass the spur road on the right leading to the Santa Catarina Spring historical marker. The road bends a little to the right. Continue along this dirt Jeep route, as directed by the "Sheep Canyon" marker sign. At just more than 2 miles, the road forks; follow the left split west toward a sign marked "Sheep Canyon Camp." At approximately 3.8 miles from the third crossing, the route dips, crossing a wide, sandy wash. Keep going past the marked right-hand

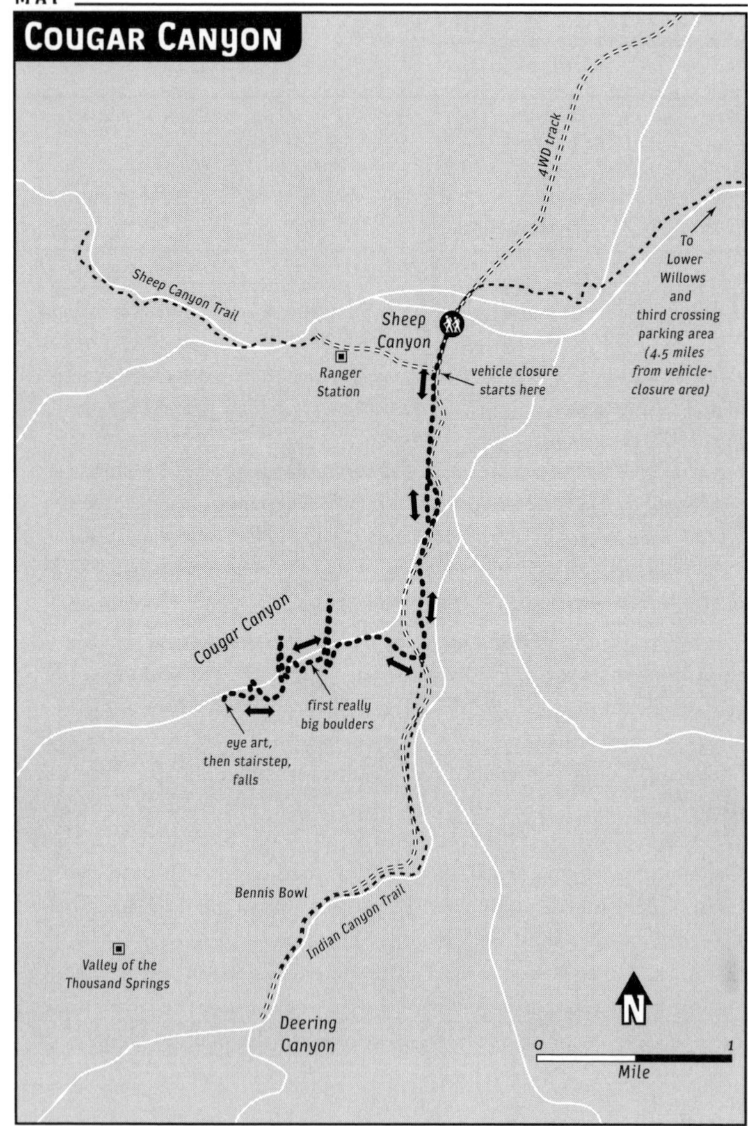
Cougar Canyon
4WD track
Sheep Canyon Trail
Sheep Canyon
To Lower Willows and third crossing parking area (4.5 miles from vehicle-closure area)
Ranger Station
vehicle closure starts here
Cougar Canyon
first really big boulders
eye art, then stairstep, falls
Bennis Bowl
Indian Canyon Trail
Valley of the Thousand Springs
Deering Canyon
N
0
1
Mile

turnoff to Sheep Canyon Primitive Camp at 4 miles. Go southwest, as directed on the marker pole, toward Indian and Cougar canyons. Another 0.1 mile brings you to a vehicle-closure sign. If you've driven, park your four-wheel drive here. If on foot, take heart: the monotonous hike across mostly flat desert, perhaps dodging the dust clouds left by speeding Jeeps, is about to end—replaced by a quiet trek into pristine desert.

Head south on the foot trail, where you may see mountain-lion prints alongside those left by hikers' boots. Cougar Canyon's name is appropriate since all of the canyon is cougar habitat, but according to Diana Lindsay's book *Anza-Borrego A to Z*, the canyon was first named Krueger Canyon, after George S. Krueger, a state-park supporter.

Make your way along the path lined with sweet-scented desert lavender, perhaps spotting birds' nests or their inhabitants. Always watch for movement, keeping safe from startled snakes or catching sight of a wily coyote disappearing, ghostlike, into the brush. Water may be present in the creek bed to your left, gurgling the opposite direction as you walk. At 0.7 miles from the vehicle-closure sign, a marker pole heralds your right turn into Cougar Canyon. From here, you'll head gradually uphill on easy

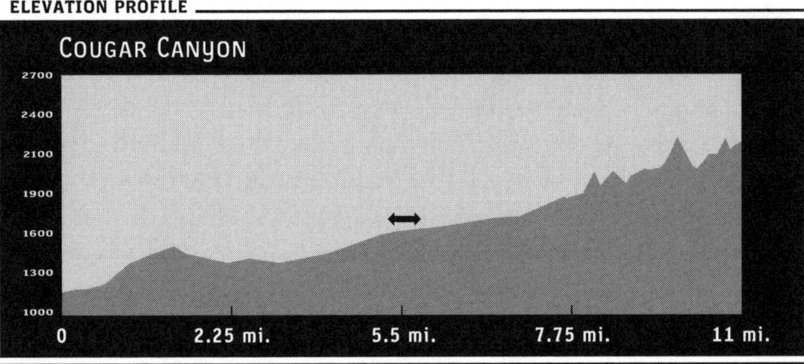

terrain for the first half mile or so, perhaps pausing to watch a flock of startled quail.

If you've moved directly upstream, approximately 0.5 miles into the canyon you'll come to a lovely spot where water sprays from several openings between massive, piled boulders. These same boulders, though, make the path ahead difficult. Work your way to the right and left, crossing the stream and climbing boulders as necessary in order to hike slowly up the canyon. Take the snail's pace as a gift that allows you to enjoy the lush surroundings.

Do you like the sound of dribbling water? Or do you prefer a low gurgle? In Cougar Canyon, you can have your pick: splatter, sprinkle, tinkle, babble, spray, or gush. Actually, those are just a few of the words that describe the variety of waterfalls you'll encounter on this gorgeous wilderness hike. You'd need a thesaurus to come up with every descriptive word, here in a place where nature has provided a staggering abundance of water falling, misting, splashing and spattering in every possible way.

On my early-spring visits to Cougar Canyon, I've encountered red-spotted toads by the hundreds. The small, pale, gray-brown toads have reddish spots and are about the size of two large almonds. Be aware of the toad's natural defense mechanism—poison secreted from glands behind each eye. The toxin causes inflammation in the mouth of a predatory animal. If you touch a toad, the poison may get on your hands, and you could easily rub it into your eyes, nose, and mouth and suffer these same symptoms; it also sometimes causes nausea and heart palpitations. Wash your hands after handling. Or better yet, observe the toads in their natural habitat but don't touch.

At about 1.3 miles, you'll find an interesting piece of rock art—an eye, painted on the eastern face of a huge boulder to the left of the stream. The creation isn't Native American, or ancient in any way: painted by a visitor to the canyon some 40 years ago. A big, soft sandbar makes this a wonderfully relaxing spot to sit and reflect or rest. Climbing much farther up the canyon becomes close to impossible, so turning around not too far past the eye is logical. Do go another 0.1 mile, though, where a beautiful stairstep falls seems the crowning glory to this beautiful hike.

If you've decided to camp, find a nice, flat spot that isn't so close to the stream that you disturb wild creatures seeking a cool drink in the night. Trek back to a wide spot you scoped out on the way in. If you've come for a day hike, give yourself plenty of daylight to get out of the canyon—and back to the third crossing if you've hoofed it all the way. You'll want to enjoy the waterfalls on your way out and pick your way sensibly over the boulders you climbed heading in. This sort of rough terrain is especially dangerous in low or no light.

Directions: From Borrego Springs, drive east on Palm Canyon Drive and turn left on DiGiorgio Road. Drive 5 miles till the pavement ends; then continue on the dirt road for another 5.6 miles to the large turnout on the left, just prior to the third crossing. If you cannot or choose not to drive all the way to this point, park at the first or second crossing, adding appropriate mileage to the hike (see the Coyote Canyon Introduction, page 52). In a four-wheel drive, it's possible to begin the hike 4 miles from the third crossing at the vehicle-closure sign—cutting this hike by 8 miles round trip.

GPS Coordinates	9 COUGAR CANYON
UTM Zone (WGS84)	11S
Easting	548672
Northing	3691851
Latitude–Longitude	N 33° 21' 53.2336"
	W 116° 28' 36.5284"

10 Indian Canyon

SCENERY: ☆☆☆☆	DISTANCE: *3.6–11.6 miles round trip*
DIFFICULTY: ☆☆☆	HIKING TIME: *3.5–8 hours*
TRAIL CONDITION: ☆☆	OUTSTANDING FEATURES: *Continuous stream; riparian habitat; quiet, open desert; beautiful views*
SOLITUDE: ☆☆☆☆	
CHILDREN: ☆	

A daylong hike from the parking area at the third crossing, or a shorter foray if your four-wheel drive can make it to the vehicle closure just past Sheep Canyon Primitive Camp. Whichever you choose, Indian Canyon is a fairly flat trek through open desert. A constant stream offers willow and tamarisk thickets and an amphibious chorus.

OPTIONS: *Camp almost anywhere in Indian Canyon. With its off-the-beaten-path location, you'll find solitude under the stars. The dense night quiet is interrupted only by the orchestra of frogs that serenade you.*

From the parking area just before the third crossing (see the Coyote Canyon Introduction, page 52), turn left and cross the stream, pass by the entrance to Lower Willows, and continue up the steep, rocky hill heading west. The rocky uphill section continues for about 0.66 miles before the road begins a gradual descent. On foot or by four-wheel drive, continue west on the Jeep road. It's about 1.5 miles till you pass the spur road on the right leading to the Santa Catarina Spring historical marker. The road bends a little to the right. Continue along this dirt Jeep route, as directed by the "Sheep Canyon" marker sign. At just more than 2 miles, the road forks; follow the left split west toward a sign marked "Sheep Canyon Camp." At approximately 3.8 miles from the third crossing, the route dips, crossing a wide, sandy wash. Keep going past the marked right-hand turnoff to Sheep Canyon Primitive Camp at 4 miles. Go southwest as directed on the marker pole, toward Indian and Cougar canyons. Another 0.1 mile brings you to a vehicle-closure sign. If you've driven, park

INDIAN CANYON

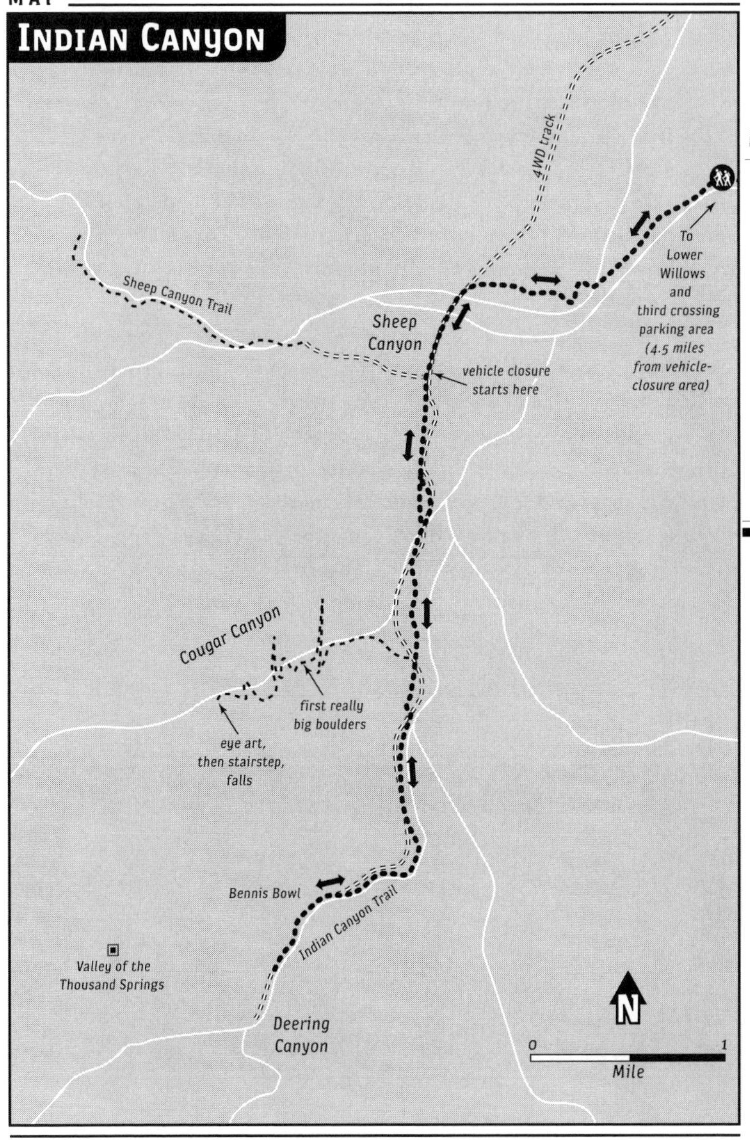

your four-wheel drive here. If on foot, take heart. Your monotonous hike along the Jeep road, perhaps dodging clouds left by four-wheel drives, is about to end—replaced by a quiet trek into pristine desert.

Head south on the foot trail (for more detail about this portion of the hike, see the Cougar Canyon write-up, page 65), passing the Cougar Canyon marker and continuing south. Past this point, the trail narrows. For most of the hike, the stream will be on your left. Soft breezes spread the scent of desert lavender. The bushes' pale-green leaves and delicate lavender blooms add a soft fringe that blurs the harsher lines of the rocky desert landscape.

About 1.4 miles past the vehicle-closure sign, the trail bends right (west). Cross back and forth across the stream on flattish rocks as needed. A fairly steady trail runs along the right of the stream, but you'll see narrow footpaths snaking around and along both sides—the obvious efforts of other hikers to find or forge a path. Some of these paths lead through tangles of feathery tamarisk that become thick to the point of turning back. Others come to dead ends at deeper, wider stream spots. You may find yourself on a trial-and-error mission to discover the most consistent path, but it's all an adventure. Indian

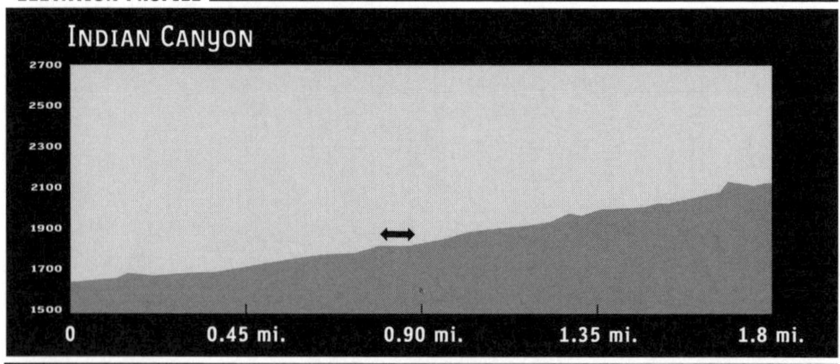

Canyon is quiet and pretty. Enjoy stream nooks where the water eddies and spills into a forest of sturdy reeds, or trickles into serene pools covered in bright-green duckweed. Your feet may get muddy.

At 1.7 miles past the vehicle-closure sign, you'll come to a fork of sorts, centered by a single palm at the end of a narrow ridge. This is where I most often turn around (and is the end of the measurement for this write-up). However, from this point, you can work your way a rugged 0.66 miles west to the Valley of a Thousand Springs. There, sycamores grow and wildlife prints are common around the stream. Or you can continue 0.5 miles south to the mouth of smaller Deering Canyon. Or simply climb up onto the ridge beyond the palm for a fantastic view back down into the desert valley. If you're not up for more hiking nor the climb, no worries—you still get a fantastic view on your way back. As you emerge from the area dense with tamarisk and willow, the valley framed by surrounding mountains comes into view.

Directions: From Borrego Springs, drive east on Palm Canyon Drive and turn left on DiGiorgio Road. Drive 5 miles till the pavement ends, then continue on the dirt road for another 5.6 miles to the large turnout on the left, just prior to the third crossing. If you cannot or choose not to drive all the way to this point, park at the first or second crossing, adding appropriate mileage to the hike (see the Coyote Canyon Introduction, page 52). In a four-wheel drive, it's possible to begin the hike 4 miles from the third crossing at the vehicle-closure sign—cutting this hike by 8 miles round trip.

GPS Coordinates	10 INDIAN CANYON
UTM Zone (WGS84)	11S
Easting	548672
Northing	3691851
Latitude–Longitude	N 33° 21' 53.2336"
	W 116° 28' 36.5284"

11 Horse Canyon

SCENERY: ☆☆☆☆
DIFFICULTY: ☆☆☆☆
TRAIL CONDITION: ☆☆☆
SOLITUDE: ☆☆☆☆
CHILDREN: ☆☆

DISTANCE: *4–6 miles round trip*
HIKING TIME: *2.5–4.5 hours*
OUTSTANDING FEATURES: *Streambed, cottonwood trees, rocky canyon views, boulders, and possible wildlife*

A 4-mile out-and-back from the bottom of the Turkey Track (aka the mouth of Horse Canyon), usually with water present; a 6-mile out-and-back starts at the top of the Turkey Track. This trek into a canyon inhabited until recently by wild horses offers a perspective on flowing water's effect on the environment.

OPTIONS: *Because access to this far-north corner of the Coyote Canyon region is extremely difficult, solitude reigns supreme. Backpacking into Horse Canyon (or surrounding canyons) allows for a remote outback experience. Packing into intersecting White Wash Canyon (see page 78) is a similar yet more distant experience. Surrounding canyons each have their own natural charm. Nance, to the west, hooks into a leg of the Pacific Crest Trail. Other canyons include Tule, to the southwest, and Alder and Salvador to the southeast. You might also head into the Upper Willows areas, perhaps visiting the Anza Monument, erected to honor an infant once believed to be the first non–Native American child born in California. For a more ambitious experience, consider a drop-off at the top of the Turkey Track and arrange for a pickup two to four days later near Lower Willows (after you've explored to your heart's content). Although 3.5 central miles of Coyote Canyon are permanently closed to vehicle traffic, backpackers, bicyclists, and horseback riders can see the route through—enjoying the park's open camping policy as they go.*

If you've left your four-wheel drive at the top of the Turkey Track, be sure to take your time walking down the steep Anza Ridge overlooking Nance Canyon, which gapes open below. By going slowly, perhaps stopping to peer down for movement or to enjoy the brushstroke view of water-molded sand or the pale-green and ochre

MAP

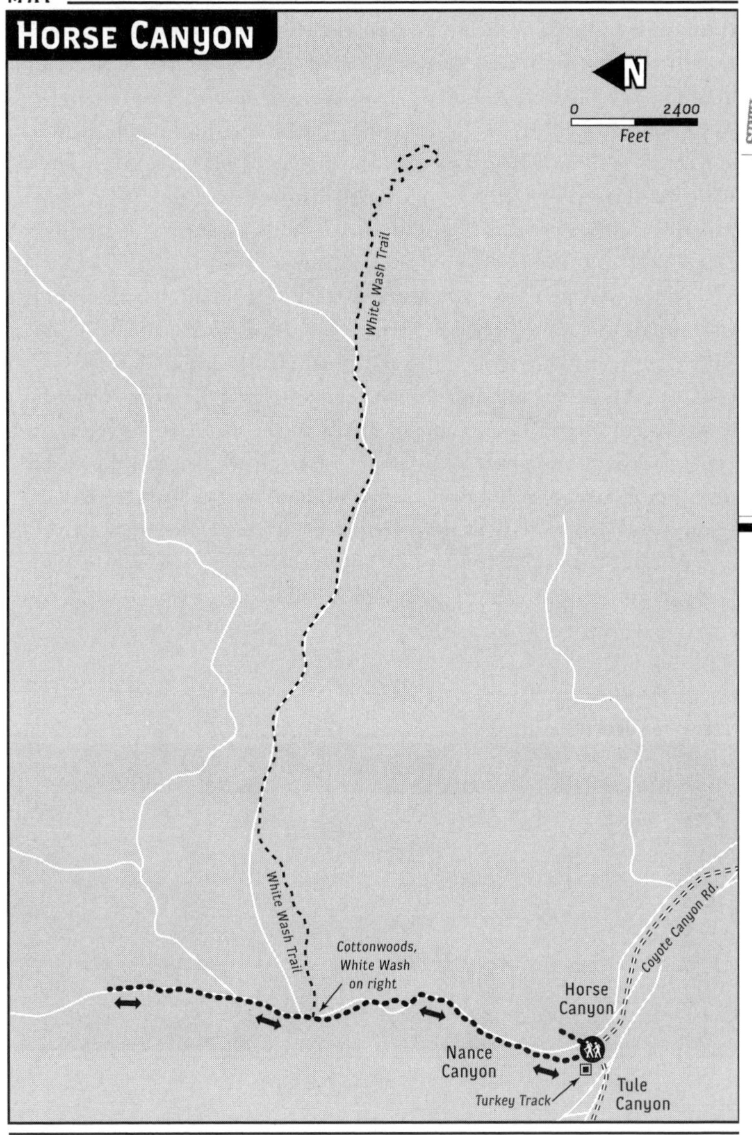

Horse Canyon
N
0
2400
Feet
White Wash Trail
White Wash Trail
Cottonwoods, White Wash on right
Horse Canyon
Coyote Canyon Rd.
Nance Canyon
Turkey Track
Tule Canyon

vegetation, you won't miss the sounds of nature. Quails run by the thousands in this remote area, their calls echoing up the canyon walls and drifting, distant and warped, to your ears above. If you know the area's recent history, you may pause, wondering if that's the neigh of horses you hear from down below. It won't be, but until recently you might well have heard or seen the beautiful wild creatures. Horse Canyon derived its name from domestic horses that escaped nearby ranches nearly a century ago, then bred, multiplying into a sizable herd. In 2003, the park removed the horses.

At the bottom of the steep turkey-track ridge road, head northeast (a compass will come in handy here). The primitive dirt roadway passes Tule Canyon on the right. Cross the stream (often an ill-defined trickle at this point) to enter the wide gap of Horse Canyon, stretching to the north where Nance Canyon opens on the west. A wide Jeep route follows the streambed. In a four-wheel drive, you could possibly drive a mile or more, but don't count on it—large sandbars, tree trunks, and debris make evident the power of heavily flowing water.

About 1.3 miles from the bottom of the ridge road, White Wash Canyon comes in on the right at a grove of shady cottonwoods. From

ELEVATION PROFILE

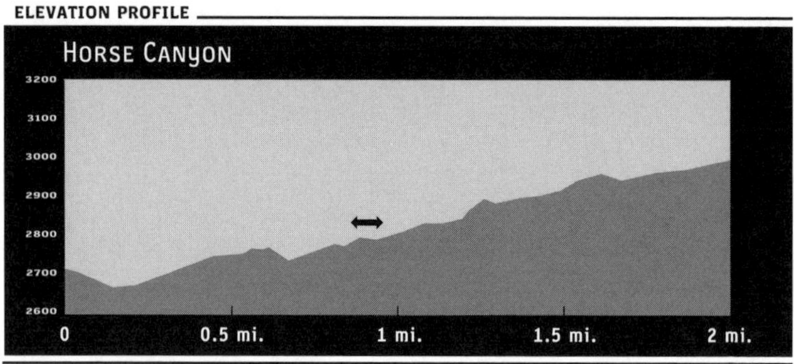

this point, easily follow the stream another 0.7 miles (or farther if you desire), enjoying the quiet in this wide rift framed by mountains. Horse Canyon can be particularly beautiful on an overcast day, when fingers of golden sun break through blanketing clouds and cast a glow on surrounding mountains. But be aware of unexpected storms. This area is remote; don't get caught in this sometimes-raging streambed. And navigating the steep section to the top of the Turkey Track could be especially dangerous in stormy weather.

Directions: Take CA 371 to the town of Anza. Turn right (south) on Kirby Road, which is 1.5 miles east of the town center. After 1 mile, Kirby Road turns left and becomes Wellman Road, which heads east. Another mile brings you to Terwilliger Road, where you must turn right (south). Drive approximately 4 miles, passing by the Anza RV resort, and turn left on Coyote Canyon Road. After about 1.6 miles, turn right to continue on Coyote Canyon Road, now dirt. You'll pass some homesites, then, at approximately 3.5 miles, a sign for Anza-Borrego Desert State Park. It's about 8 miles on Coyote Canyon Road to the park gate. The first 2 miles of road are rough, but not too difficult for four-wheel-drive vehicles. After that, the road reaches what's considered the topmost part of the Turkey Track, which is the merging point for stream flow from Horse, Tule, and Nance canyons—the three "toes" of a huge (and, of course, imaginary) Turkey Track. A wide, flat turnout on the left offers a stop-and-get-out point for those not wanting to continue down the steep, rugged road. Sharp turns over extremely rocky and pitted terrain that overhangs gaping Nance Canyon way below cause pause. It's approximately 0.5 miles down this steep, rugged section known as the Anza Ridge, then another 0.5 miles or so (northwest) to the mouth of Horse Canyon.

GPS Coordinates	11 HORSE CANYON
UTM Zone (WGS84)	11S
Easting	542439
Northing	3703432
Latitude–Longitude	N 33° 28' 10.2191" W 116° 32' 35.7690"

12 White Wash

Scenery: ★★★★
Difficulty: ★★★
Trail Condition: ★★★
Solitude: ★★★★★
Children: ★
Distance: *7.8 miles round trip*

Hiking Time: *4.5–5.5 hours*
Outstanding Features: *Wide, rocky wash leading to higher desert features such as manzanita and piñon pine, possible wildlife spotting, and an awesome Clark Valley view*

An out-and-back hike from the cottonwoods in Horse Canyon, treading through the rocky wash named for its salt-and-pepper granitic rocks and sediment. The wash narrows and climbs approximately 1,200 feet for a fantastic view of Clark Valley.

OPTIONS: *Because access to this far-north corner of the Coyote Canyon region is extremely difficult, solitude reigns supreme. Backpacking into Horse Canyon, White Wash, or surrounding canyons and washes allows for a remote outback experience. Other area canyons each have their own natural charm. Nance, to the west, hooks into a leg of the Pacific Crest Trail. Other canyons include Tule, to the southwest, or Alder and Salvador to the southeast. Or head down into the Upper Willows areas, perhaps visiting the Anza Monument, erected to honor an infant once believed the first non–Native American child born in California. For a more ambitious experience, consider a drop-off at the top of the Turkey Track, and arrange for a pickup two to four days later near Lower Willows (after you've explored to your heart's content). Though 3.5 central miles of Coyote Canyon are permanently closed to vehicles, backpackers, bicyclists, and horseback riders can see the route through—enjoying the park's open-camping policy as they go.*

The official White Wash trailhead begins at the junction of Horse Canyon and White Wash, where cottonwoods shade the trail. To get to the trailhead, see the Horse Canyon profile (page 74).

Start by heading east into the wash from Horse Canyon. Note the black-and-white-speckled granitics and their gravelly sand. When viewed as a whole, the scene looks more white than black. It's interesting how the eye blocks the darker color, focusing instead on the light, so the entire wash looks white—hence the name. The gain in elevation begins immediately but is gradual at the outset.

MAP

White Wash

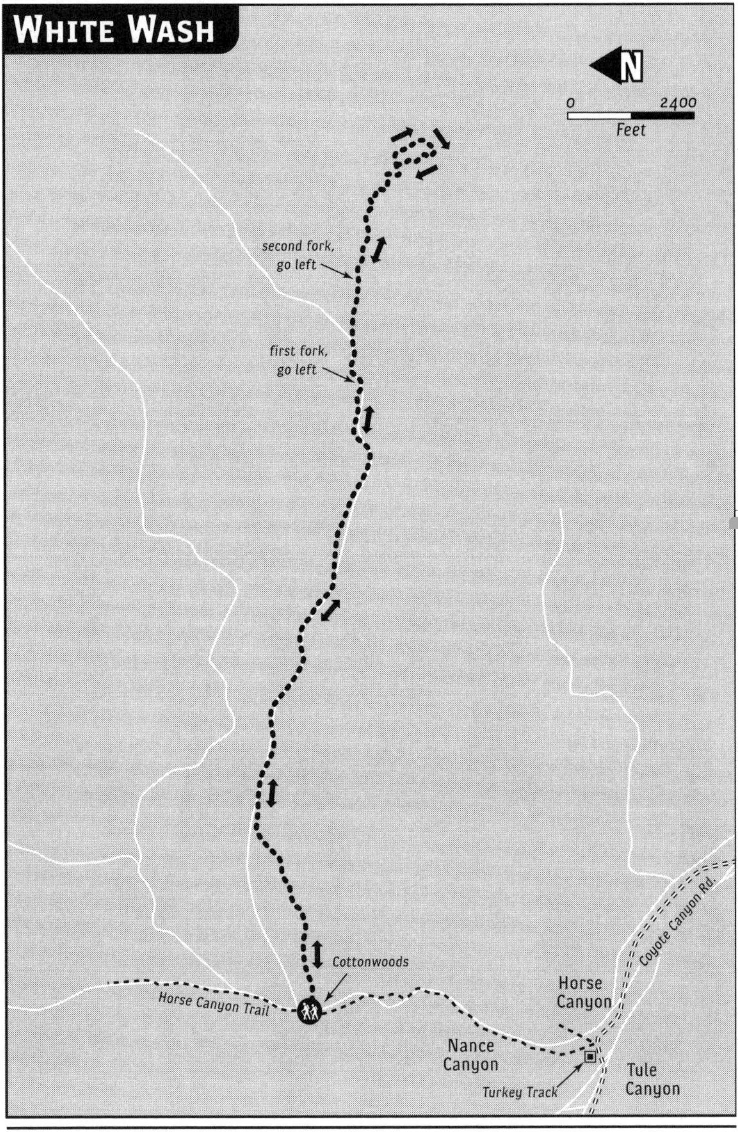

N
0 2400
Feet
second fork, go left
first fork, go left
Cottonwoods
Horse Canyon Trail
Horse Canyon
Coyote Canyon Rd.
Nance Canyon
Turkey Track
Tule Canyon

At approximately 1.3 miles, the wash narrows, and you'll begin to see small pinecones littering the wash. The cones fall from piñon trees growing atop the south side of the ridge. The silence in this isolated wash is enhanced by the hush of wind drafts similar to that in the valleys surrounding Whale Peak (see the Blair Valley Introduction, page 93). Birdcalls also punctuate the air, particularly the twisting notes of hummingbirds. Scan the ridge for movement. You might get lucky and see bighorn sheep, whose prints are plentiful in White Wash.

The wash narrows more at about 2.2 miles, and big boulders begin to encroach, requiring you to climb over them in a few spots. Although climbing elevation thus far has been evenly spread, the increasing presence of manzanita trees now confirms the gain of nearly 1,000 feet.

At miles 2.5 and 2.9, small ridges blocking the center of the wash require you to choose the left fork in the splitting trail, which grows narrower and narrower. The route becomes little more than a two- to three-foot gulch at times.

At 3 miles and an approximate 3,800-foot elevation, piñon pines begin growing alongside the trail. At around 3.4 miles, the gulch heads to the left, then quickly comes to a dead end of sorts. Your only options will be a very steep climb to a high ridge on the left or a shorter climb on the right. Choose the shorter climb out of the

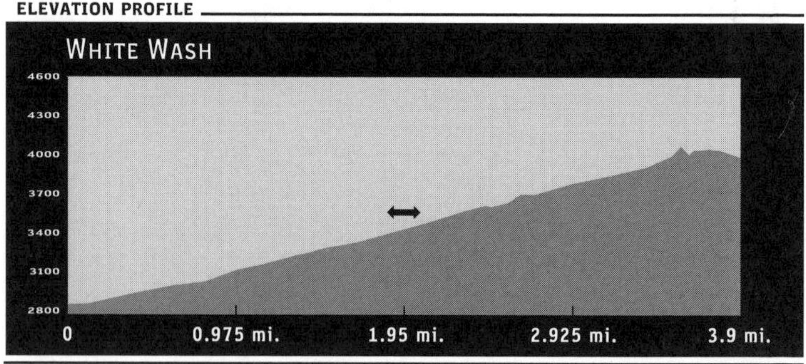

gulch, then along a narrow ridge, heading southeast to a point overlooking Clark Valley. The ridgetop moves southwest for a short distance, still offering a gorgeous view into the valley. At mile 3.6, you'll see a short, semisteep gulch on the right. You could retrace your steps along the ridge back to the trail from this high point or move carefully down this new gulch, heading northwest on your right. This hooks back to the lower route.

Whether you hike out of White Wash the same day or camp in one of the many beautiful spots in this remote region, savor the splendor of solitude in nature. Take note of the scents and sounds, memorizing these gifts for earthy recall after returning to your everyday life.

Directions: Take CA 371 to the town of Anza. Turn right (south) on Kirby Road (1.5 miles east of the town center). After 1 mile, Kirby Road turns left and becomes Wellman Road, which heads east. Another mile brings you to Terwilliger Road, where you must turn right (south). Drive approximately 4 miles, passing by the Anza RV resort, and turn left on Coyote Canyon Road. After about 1.6 miles, turn right to continue on Coyote Canyon Road, now dirt. You'll pass some homesites and, at approximately 3.5 miles, a sign for Anza-Borrego Desert State Park. It's about 8 miles on Coyote Canyon Road to the park gate. The first 2 miles of road are rough but not too difficult for four-wheel drives. After that, the road reaches what's considered the topmost part of the Turkey Track, which is the merging point for stream flow from Horse, Tule, and Nance canyons—the three "toes" of a huge (and of course, imaginary) Turkey Track. A wide, flat turnout on the left offers a stop-and-get-out point for those not wanting to continue down the steep, rugged road. Sharp turns over extremely rocky and pitted terrain that overhangs gaping Nance Canyon way below cause pause. It's approximately 0.5 miles down this steep, rugged section known as the Anza Ridge, then another 0.5 miles or so (northwest) to the mouth of Horse Canyon. White Horse Wash is on the right, 1.3 miles into Horse Canyon.

GPS Coordinates	**12 WHITE WASH**
UTM Zone (WGS84)	**11S**
Easting	**542439**
Northing	**3703432**
Latitude–Longitude	**N 33° 28' 10.2191"**
	W 116° 32' 35.7690"

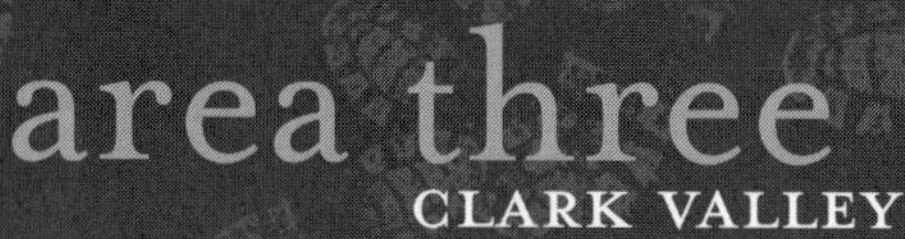

3

area three

CLARK VALLEY

Many
consider
the
desert
dry
and desolate
but
secret oases
cool
waterfalls
interesting
animals
and
a wide
array of
adaptive
vegetation
wait
quietly
to refresh
adventurous
souls

AREA 3: CLARK VALLEY

Introduction

Clark Valley, named for a pair of brothers who saw the value of this area as cattle land, lies between Coyote Mountain and the Santa Rosa Mountains. Faults in this area grew the Santa Rosa Mountains and formed the basin of Clark Dry Lake (dry lakes have no drainage). I've outlined a 10-mile canyon loop that, in my opinion, is the best hiking in this area. Other adventures you might embark on include trekking up Coyote Mountain from its east side, starting at the mountain's base just west of Clark Dry Lake. Also, a short view hike begins at the Pegleg Smith monument, which is found where County Route S22 meets Henderson Canyon Road. Pegleg Smith, born in 1801, was a gold prospector—and a storyteller. Apparently, he had quite the penchant for spinning lost-mine tales, and to honor his talent, an annual competition is held to this day. The Pegleg Smith Liar's Contest takes place at the monument in early April.

13 Butler Canyon– Rockhouse Canyon Loop

SCENERY: ☆☆☆	DISTANCE: *9.6 miles round trip*
DIFFICULTY: ☆☆☆	HIKING TIME: *6–6.5 hours*
TRAIL CONDITION: ☆☆☆	OUTSTANDING FEATURES: *Canyon views, interesting rock formations, open desert/desert wash, and a hidden spring*
SOLITUDE: ☆☆☆☆	
CHILDREN: ☆☆	

A wonderful day hike with fairly easy terrain, this long loop leads through the twisting upper end of Butler Canyon and across open desert before approaching a precipice overlooking Rockhouse Canyon. You'll pass near a Cahuilla Indian ruin site, so you could spend extra time exploring there, then take the narrow path down into Rockhouse Canyon and loop back to your car.

OPTION: *The wide-open space between upper Butler Canyon and Rockhouse Canyon makes for an interesting overnight experience. At night, the star-studded sky seems to go on forever. An easy backpack into this loop's midpoint leaves an equally easy finish for the following day—after rising with the sun and perhaps cooking over a campfire (in a metal container, of course, as park rules dictate).*

You could take the loop from either direction, but I prefer Butler Canyon—the left-hand leg—at the outset. At just under 1 mile, the dirt road ends. Continue northwest into the center of the narrowing canyon, climbing over some boulder stands but staying on a relatively identifiable and continuous footpath. Marvel at the canyon walls, varnished a deep desert bronze (the effect of microscopic bacteria). Butler Canyon is reminiscent of old Hollywood westerns, the terrain perfect for ridgetop lookouts and surprise ambushes.

After less than 2 miles, you'll reach a wide wash that continues northwest for another 2 miles. At 4.2 miles, the wash bends to the right (northeast). After another 0.5 miles, the canyon opens. Make

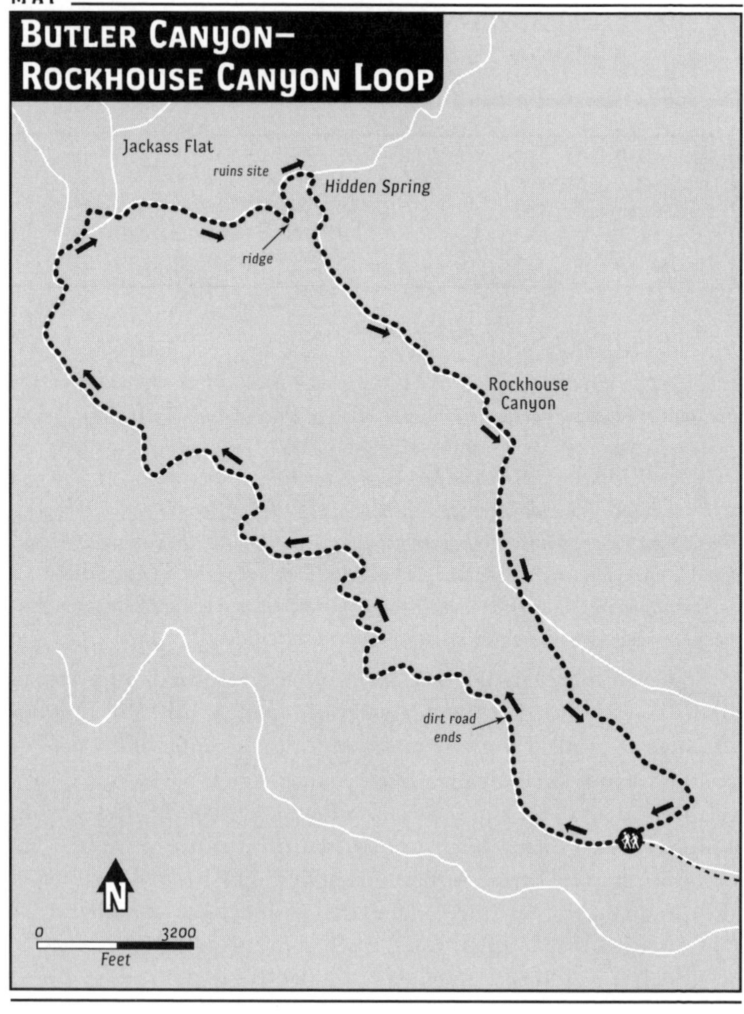

Butler Canyon–
Rockhouse Canyon Loop
Jackass Flat
ruins site
Hidden Spring
ridge
Rockhouse
Canyon
dirt road
ends
N
0
3200
Feet

sure you turn more to the right now (east) rather than continuing north into Jackass Flat. The flat land between Butler and Rockhouse canyons was named for wild burros that once roamed here, though the burros have been gone since the early 1970s.

Moving east, you'll begin to see more ocotillo. The incidence of cholla cactus also thickens, but not so much as to be an issue for hikers. After another mile (5.8 miles from the trailhead), you'll come to the ridge overlooking Rockhouse Canyon, which appears rather suddenly, so be careful not to let children run ahead. If you have time, explore a little before going down the path into the canyon. Above Rockhouse Canyon is a Cahuilla Indian ruins site. You might be able to spot evidence of the natives' lives here in this protected site, in the form of piled rocks (for their fires or houses), but identification isn't easy for the untrained eye.

Whether or not you search for ruins, be sure to pause a bit to absorb the view of Rockhouse Canyon. There's something mesmerizing about this deep gorge etched rather suddenly into the land. Perhaps this is one reason the Indians chose this site. When you're ready to move on, look for the narrow, worn footpath leading down into the canyon, which first heads north, then bends east. Be careful—this path may be slippery in spots due to loose rocks and soil.

At the bottom, you'll need to backtrack (left) about 50 feet to see Hidden Spring, which is not much more than a bit of moisture covered in vegetation. The spring lives up to its name. You'd likely miss it entirely if you didn't know of its presence or perhaps see bees hovering and realize what they're after.

From the spring, turn back around and head southwest into Rockhouse Canyon. Meander a little in the wide path, enjoying this last leg of the loop back to your car, along the canyon framed by sandstone and conglomerate walls.

ELEVATION PROFILE

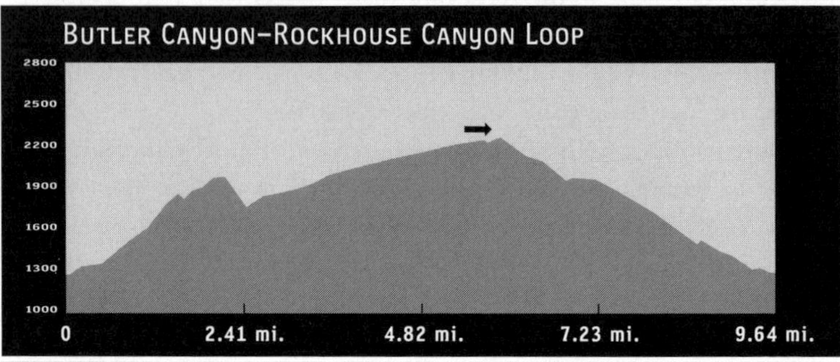

Directions: From Borrego Springs, drive east on Palm Canyon Drive. Continue almost 6 miles before the road veers left, becoming Pegleg Road. Drive on Pegleg for 8 miles to Rockhouse Canyon Trail and turn right. The pavement ends after several hundred yards, but continue on the dirt road (four-wheel drive recommended but not always necessary for high-clearance vehicles). After 1.3 miles, you will come to a split in the road. Bear left and continue, passing Clark Dry Lake on your right. After 3.2 miles on the dirt road, pass a sand company gate and continue following the dirt road, bending right. At 8.8 miles from the Pegleg Road turnoff, you'll come to a trail marker pole where Butler and Rockhouse canyons meet. Park just off the road.

GPS Coordinates	13 BUTLER CANYON—ROCKHOUSE CANYON LOOP
UTM Zone (WGS84)	11S
Easting	558973
Northing	3694390
Latitude–Longitude	N 33° 23' 13.8346" W 116° 21' 57.3140"

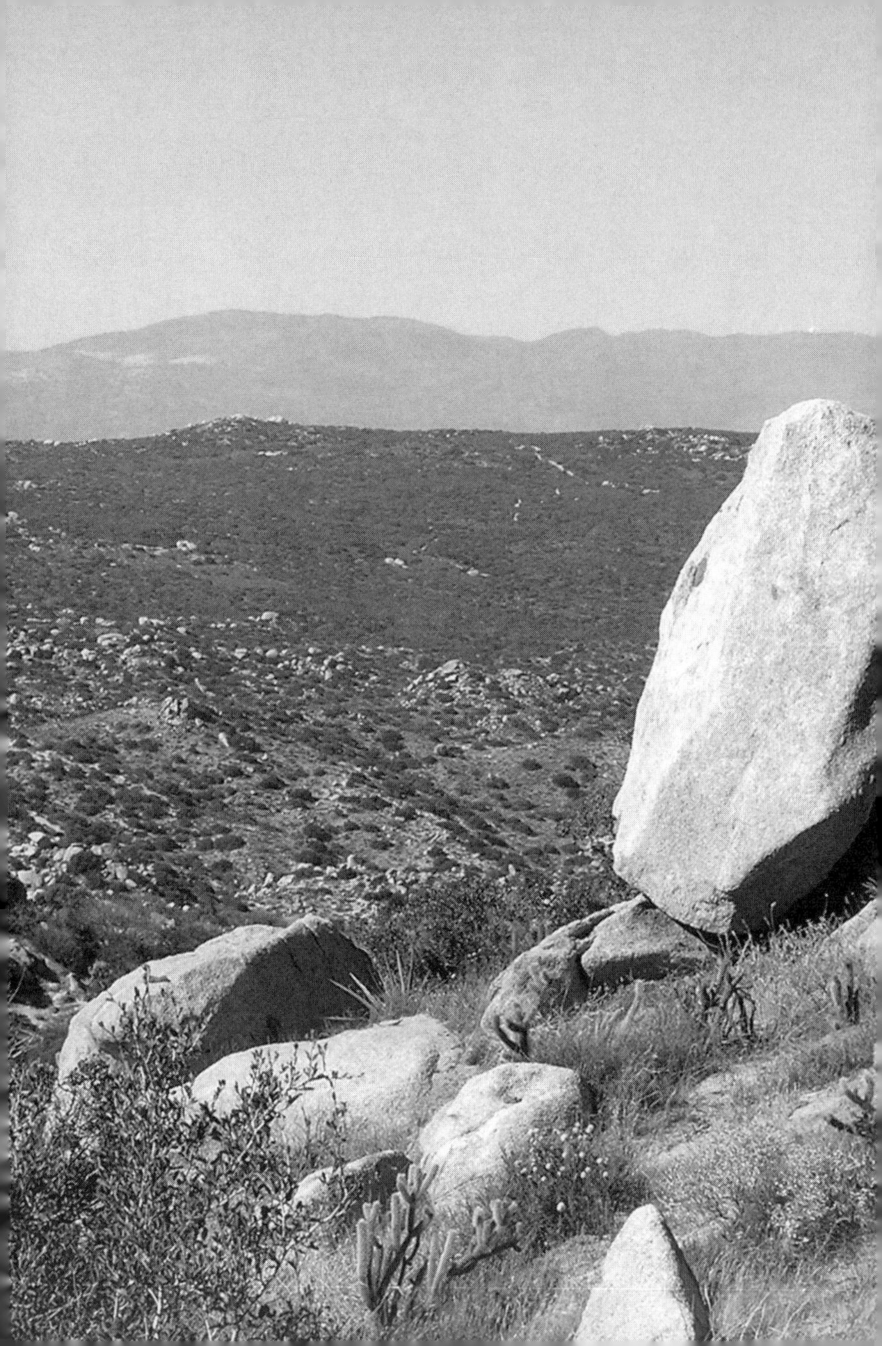

area four

BLAIR VALLEY

4

Many consider the desert dry and desolate but secret oases cool waterfalls interesting animals and a wide array of adaptive vegetation wait quietly to refresh adventurous souls

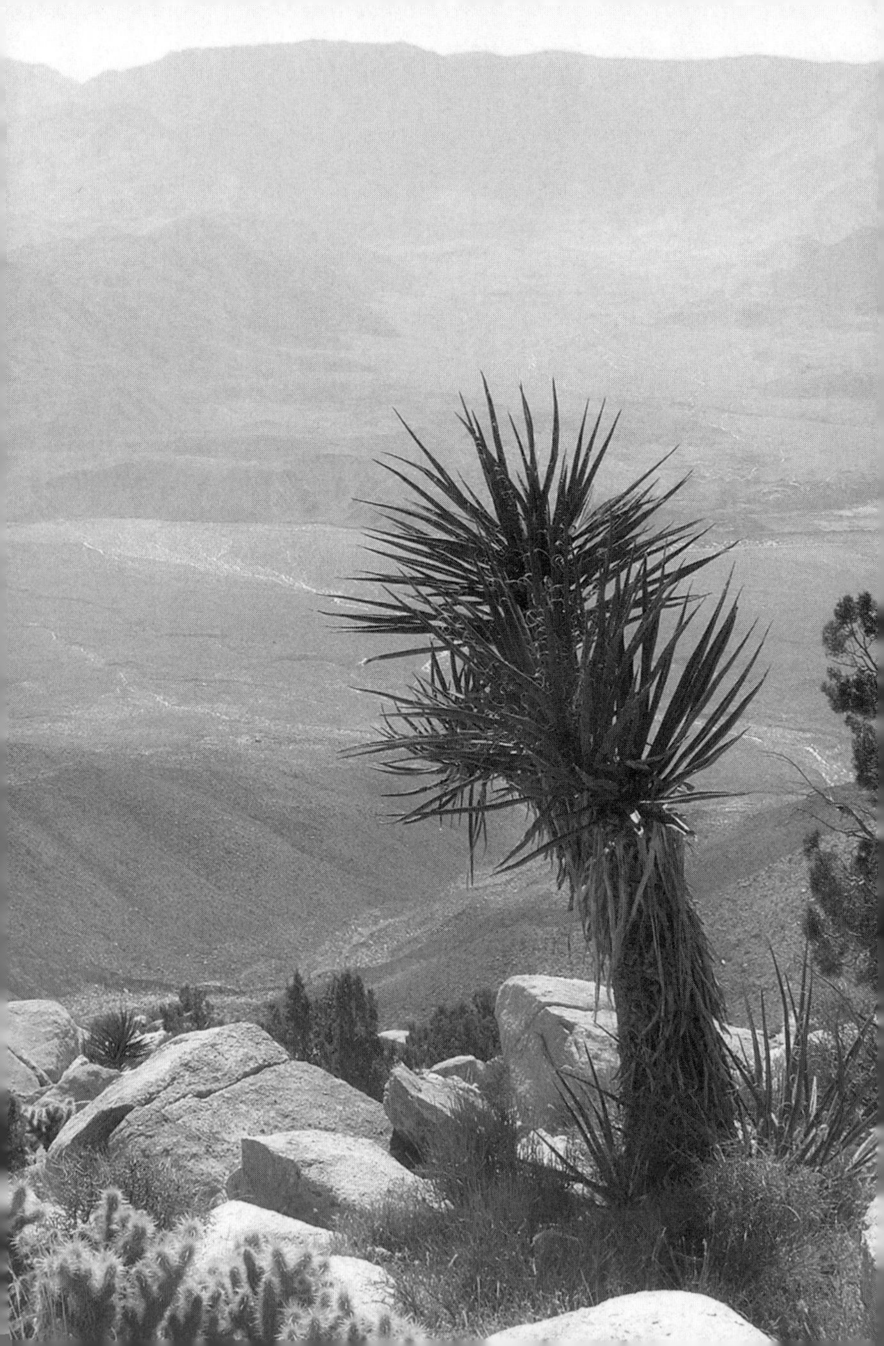

Introduction

Blair Valley is in the south of Anza-Borrego Desert State Park, between 5,633-foot Granite Mountain and 5,349-foot Whale Peak. Much of the recreational area accessed via the Blair Valley and Little Blair Valley turnoffs from County Route S2 is suitable for two-wheel-drive vehicles, contributing to the region's popularity with RV and tent campers and day visitors alike. Two of the hikes in this section, Whale Peak and Pinyon Mountain, are accessed via Pinyon Ridge Road, requiring a four-wheel-drive vehicle to reach the trailheads—or the addition of 5.7 walking miles from CR S2.

Blair Valley itself rests at an elevation of approximately 2,500 feet. The region's surrounding canyons, ridges, and peaks rise nearly a mile high and play host to changing vegetation that reflects such heights. Common desert growth such as yellow-bloomed creosote, yucca, and spiky cholla cactus gives way in stages to thorny acacia catclaw, pale-green jojoba, and more typically mountainous flora, including juniper, piñon pine, and red-wooded manzanita.

Here I've shared some of my favorite hikes, such as the colorful gorges and wide, quiet washes of the Rainbow Canyon Loop. Ponder Native American lore and daily life along the Pictograph Trail and at The Mortreros, or venture deep into the brush beside a gurgling brook along Oriflamme Canyon Trail. Poetry resides in the wind as you climb Ghost Mountain toward the remnants of the South family cabin, while gusty breezes lure you to the top of Whale Peak.

In the Blair Valley region's middle and high desert, rugged natural beauty, a dose of colorful history, and even a bit of mystery await you.

14 Pinyon Mountain

SCENERY: ★★★★
DIFFICULTY: ★★★★
TRAIL CONDITION: ★
SOLITUDE: ★★★★
CHILDREN: ★
DISTANCE: *1.2–2 miles round trip*
HIKING TIME: *2 hours*
OUTSTANDING FEATURES: *Rocky, steep trail dotted with sharp yucca leads to sweeping views of Pinyon Valley, the Salton Sea, Whale Peak, and the Santa Rosa Mountains*

Beginning at an elevation of nearly 3,900 feet at the center of Pinyon Mountain Valley and climbing to more than 4,400 feet, this hike is a brief burst over rocky terrain to an eagle's vantage point. The desert and mountain views are worth the effort.

From the trailhead parking, there are two possible routes up to the ridge. The most discernible is off to the right, edging northeast on flat ground, then northwest up an extremely steep and slippery slope. It's easier, though, on this first quick gain of close to 200 feet, to head straight or slightly to the left, more directly up to the ridge. Find others' old footholds or make your own (the steep route is less slippery from use this way, which is why I've marked the map to show this way up). Once at the ridge, the route levels out some, heading northwest and more slowly gaining the remaining 200 feet to the peak.

On your way up the ridge, you may wonder why this mountain has its name. There are few piñon (also spelled *pinyon*) pines on this, the southern side. Instead, find interestingly shaped boulders and low-growing yucca, the sharp ends of which your ankles are likely to painfully encounter. High-top hiking boots and long pants are encouraged.

Continue northwest until the ridge widens, giving way to the flattish peak. Here, you can perch on a sun-warmed boulder and enjoy the view. You'll notice more piñon pines growing on the north slope and spy the vaporous blue strip of the Salton Sea, California's largest lake, to the northeast. Whale Peak stretches out in plain view to the south from atop Pinyon Mountain.

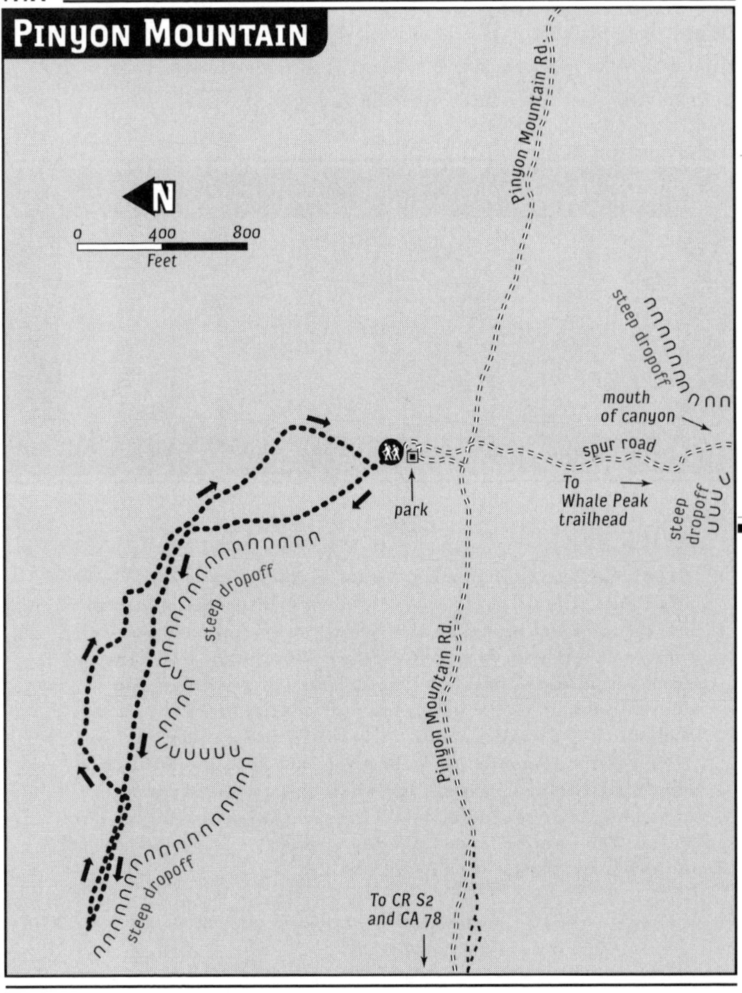
PINYON MOUNTAIN
N
0
400
800
Feet
Pinyon Mountain Rd.
steep dropoff
mouth of canyon
spur road
To Whale Peak trailhead
steep dropoff
park
steep dropoff
Pinyon Mountain Rd.
steep dropoff
To CR S2 and CA 78

To head back, either retrace your steps along the ridge and down, or venture north a bit, looping back to the ridge and then down the steeper, more evident (but slippery with loose dirt) path farther east (see map on previous page).

ELEVATION PROFILE

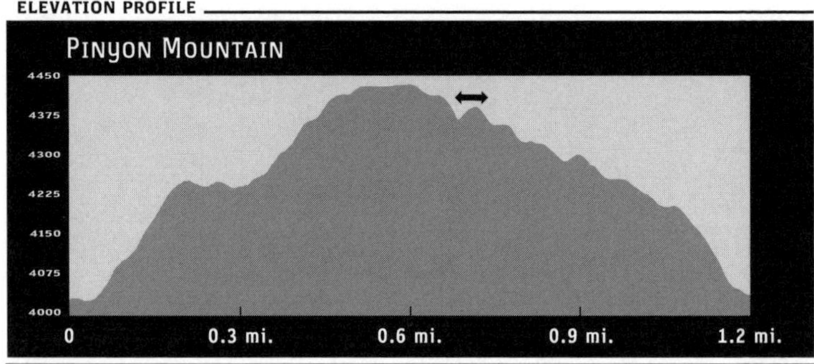

Directions: Where CA 78 meets County Route S2 (the Great Overland Route of 1849), head south on S2. At approximately 4.4 miles, note the large sign on the right marking your entrance into Anza-Borrego Desert State Park. A few feet past this, on the left, a smaller sign reads "Pinyon Mountains" and marks a dirt road (Pinyon Mountain Road). You'll need a four-wheel drive to get to the trailhead, which is 5.7 miles up this increasingly rutted and rocky road. In a regular automobile, park where you can, adding walking miles to the total distance. In your four-wheel drive, proceed east up the road, ignoring turnoffs. You'll have reached the road's crest in Pinyon Mountain Valley at 5.7 miles. Drive 0.2 miles to the turnoff on the left and park at the base of the ridge.

GPS Coordinates	14 PINYON MOUNTAIN
UTM Zone (WGS84)	11S
Easting	562251
Northing	3657168
Latitude–Longitude	N 33° 3' 4.5549"
	W 116° 19' 59.6392"

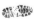

15 Whale Peak

SCENERY: ☆☆☆☆	DISTANCE: *4.5 miles round trip*
DIFFICULTY: ☆☆☆	HIKING TIME: *4–4.5 hours*
TRAIL CONDITION: ☆☆☆	OUTSTANDING FEATURES: *A series of rocky ridges lined with piñon pines; hidden valleys; sweeping breezes; panoramic views*
SOLITUDE: ☆☆☆☆	
CHILDREN: ☆☆	

Beginning at an elevation of 3,896 feet in the center of Pinyon Mountain Valley, this hike seems more like a trek through a mountain pine forest than a visit to the desert. Educationally enchanting, the area gives hikers a broader view of what desert land can really be like. A mixture of short but steep ascents and valleys, the trail culminates at the top of Whale Peak, which, at 5,250 feet, is just short of a mile high. The wide, flattish peak top is like an island set in the sky and offers panoramic views.

OPTIONS: *Make this a day hike, or backpack in and camp near the base of Whale Peak (or at some other point along the route) for an evening of serenity in this beautiful wilderness.*

If you've parked near the main dirt road, trek south across sandy, cholla-spotted desert toward the narrow canyon opening. From there, head south, with a slight westerly angle, directly into the divide. Continue on this obvious route up-canyon, using handholds to climb boulders as needed (nothing too difficult). The blue, gray, or gauzy, cloud-dotted sky is a soaring strip above, the point at which you're aiming as you climb the narrow gorge. Enjoy the scent of abundant piñon pines as you brush past them. Opening the petals of their small, brown cones to expose the nuts in late summer and early fall, the trees provide food for resident birds and mammals.

At about 0.6 miles (0.4 from the canyon mouth), the trail levels, widening into a sandy wash, which you'll follow southwest. After a short distance, take the discernible trail leading toward the ridge on

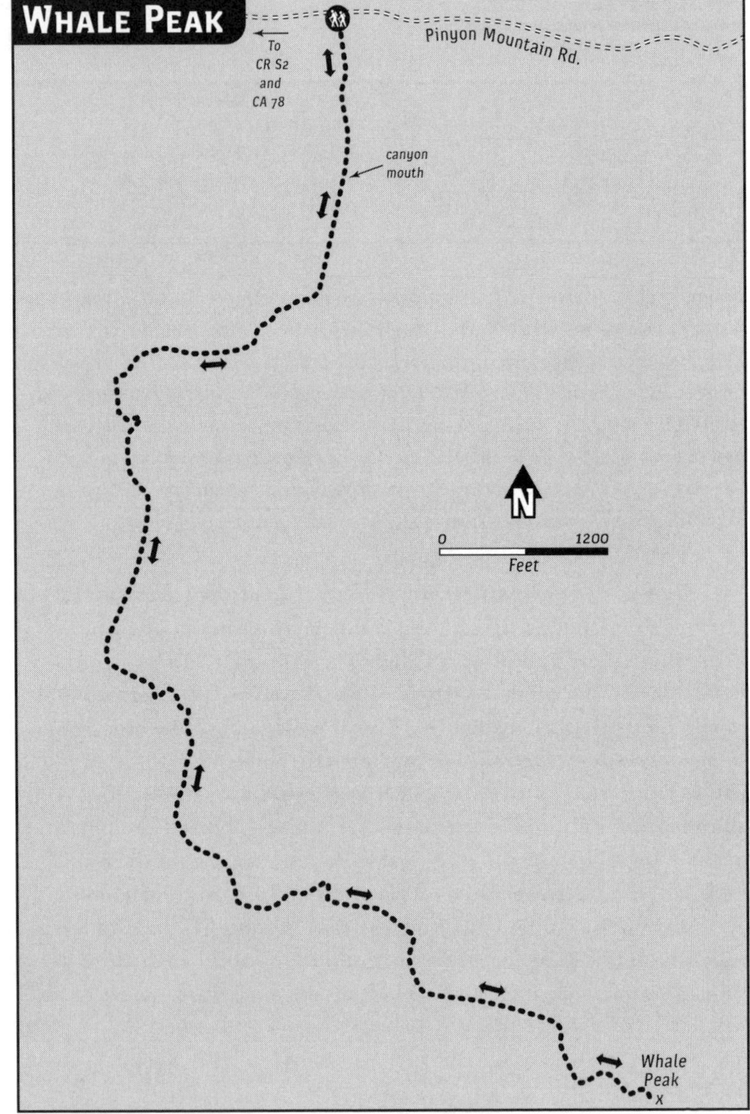

Whale Peak
To
CR S2
and
CA 78
Pinyon Mountain Rd.
canyon
mouth
N
0
1200
Feet
Whale
Peak

your left. Climb the ridge, ascending quickly. At this point, the exact route isn't as important as getting up and over, as is indicated by several rugged paths etched into the rocky soil. Continue at a slightly southwest clip, altered only by a couple of minor bends. At 0.9 miles, the trail approaches a flat expanse flanked by another ridge to the southeast (on your left). Your destination is on the other side of that formidable ridge. Bypass the climb by taking the level trail that curves decidedly more southwest (right). After about 0.2 miles on this catch-your-breath flat, the path bends left again, ascending only slightly, allowing you to save your energy for the remaining hike.

Savor the clear, pine-scented air and sweeping breezes here. You'll note the prominent growth of a variety of lichen on the rocks, evidence of the oxygen-rich air in this wilderness. The winds sweep up from the desert valleys, rustle through the pines, ruffle hair, and cool sweat-moistened skin, then dash away again, with a sound like distant waves. To the south, the Laguna Mountains come into view, rising like the long, ridged span of a gator's tail.

At just over a mile, the southeasterly route descends into a narrow, piñon-furred valley. The path ascends again, short, level stretches interspersed with short, steep climbs that top out after

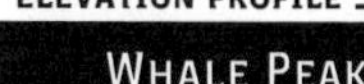

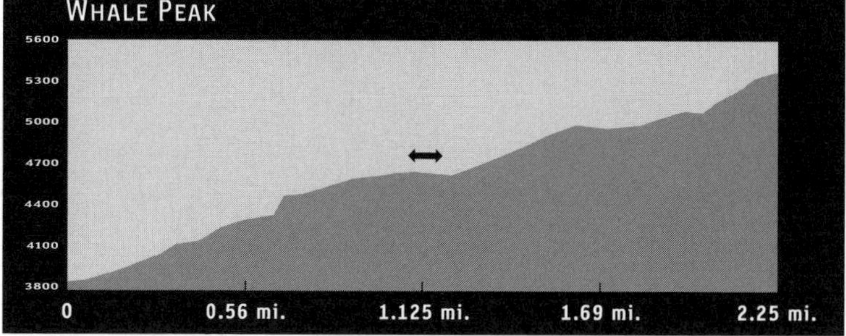

another 0.5 miles. Continue several yards across this flat section to a drop-off of sorts at the base of Whale Peak. Shaped as it's named, the peak finally comes into view ahead. You'll have traveled 1.8 miles from the main road turnout (1.6 from the canyon mouth). Move over and around boulders to the right, making your way to the southwestern base of Whale Peak. Here, a clear trail begins anew, level at first, then climbing to the peak. The path remains evident almost to the top, dwindling the last several yards, forcing you to carefully scramble up between the rocks and around dense piñon pines to reach the peak.

Whale Peak is a large, rather flat expanse covered with pines and boulders. The flat top, coupled with its growth and rocks, makes for a feeling of safety at this vantage point just under a mile in the sky. In the spring, butterflies are abundant, their flitter-flutter lending a fairytale air to this hike's endpoint.

Near the center of this island in the sky, a metal can holds a cache of hikers' notes behind a stone wall. Read through the entries, or perhaps add your own as you ponder the see-forever view.

Head back the way you came. When descending, choose your path carefully. Several trails snake their way down and around the mountain, some leading to high dead ends on boulder tops, requiring you to expend time and energy climbing back to the main path and trying again.

Directions: Where CA 78 meets County Route S2 (the Great Overland Route of 1849), head south on S2. At approximately 4.4 miles, note the large sign on the right marking your entrance into Anza-Borrego Desert State Park. A few feet past this, on the left, a smaller sign reads "Pinyon Mountains" and marks a dirt road (Pinyon Mountain Road). You'll need a four-wheel-drive vehicle to get to the trailhead, which is 5.7 miles up this increasingly rutted and rocky road. In a regular automobile, park where you can, adding walking miles to the total distance. In a four-wheel drive, proceed east up the road, ignoring turnoffs. You'll reach the road's crest in Pinyon Mountain Valley at 5.7 miles. Small turnouts allow for parking right next to the road, or drive up the 0.2-mile turnoff on the right to the opening of a narrow canyon divide, where you can also park.

GPS Coordinates	15 WHALE PEAK
UTM Zone (WGS84)	11S
Easting	563083
Northing	3656917
Latitude–Longitude	N 33° 2' 56.2314"
	W 116° 19' 27.6338"

16 Rainbow Canyon Loop

SCENERY: ☆☆☆☆
DIFFICULTY: ☆☆☆
TRAIL CONDITION: ☆☆☆
SOLITUDE: ☆☆☆☆
CHILDREN: ☆☆

DISTANCE: *8.45 miles round trip*
HIKING TIME: *3.5–4 hours*
OUTSTANDING FEATURES: *Colorful, veined rock and dry waterfalls to shimmy up and over, wood-rat nests, and open desert filled with cholla and prickly pear cacti*

Striated rock formations give this canyon its name. The path leads over natural rock slides reminiscent of a child's playground. Short climbs up slick dry waterfalls and rock shelves alternate with easy, mostly flat trail that includes a few gradual ascents. Peaceful solitude reigns for most of this trek, but there may be campers and horseback riders in Blair Valley, and you'll see cars along County Route S2.

From the parking turnout, hike along the narrow trail starting out southeast alongside S2 and moving gradually away from the road toward the canyon opening. After about 0.5 miles on this cholla-heavy route, you'll come to a fence marking private property at the park's boundary. Turn left, moving up a wide, sandy wash of flat terrain that stretches 0.25 miles, then narrows and grows rocky as the canyon walls rise on either side.

Fleshy chalk live-forever clings to the rocky canyon walls. About 0.3 miles after turning left away from the highway (0.8 miles from the trailhead), begin to make a few short shelf climbs. The colorfully swirled rock is spectacular in hues of blue and gray. Look for the clumpy nests of wood rats in high rock crevices as the trail bends right.

Continue east, encountering scraggly juniper and bushy palo verde trees. At 1.2 miles, climb a striped rock slide (dry waterfall), which is followed quickly by a few more that also require handholds. The choppy lay of the rock makes these fairly simple for agile hikers. Flat terrain then leads through the canyon, heading southeast and climbing another shelf into more sandy terrain. You'll spot lots of

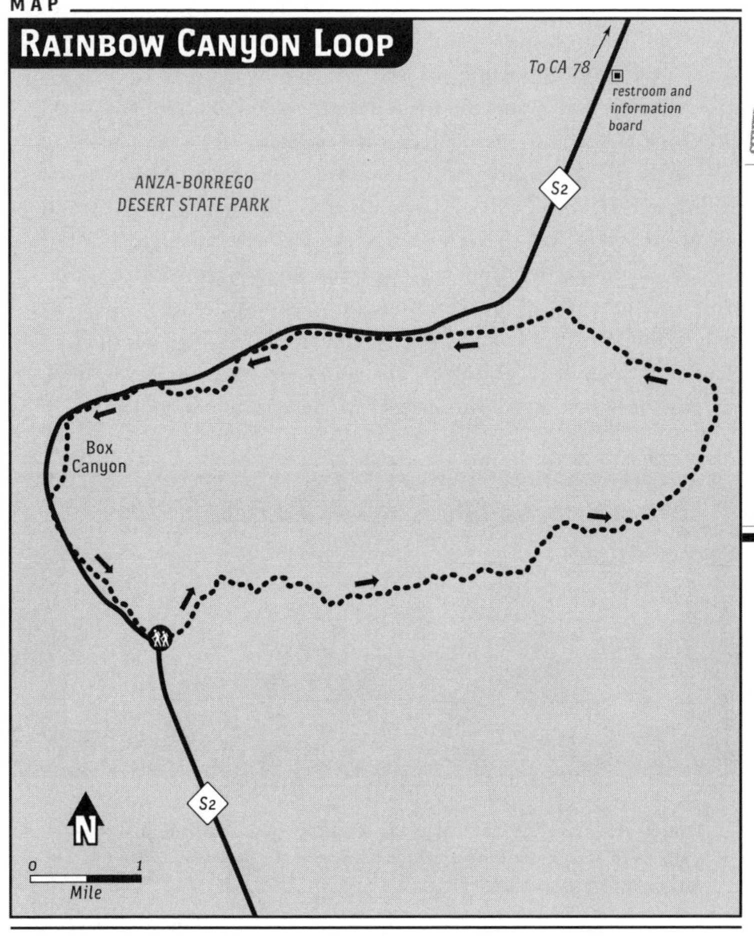

coyote scat; note the scratch marks fanning out in the sand. This is the coyote's attempt to spread his scent and better mark the territory.

When you reach a wide bowl, continue northeast on easy terrain marked by dark rock, cholla, beavertail, and spider cactus. At around

2.9 miles, climb the gentle slope out of the bowl and continue northeast. You'll soon come to sandy wash with flat terrain. At about 4.4 miles, you'll notice the hills on your left coming to an end. Turn left, moving toward S2 across the rocky desert, careful of abundant prickly pear cactus. You'll come to a Jeep road, perhaps with a few parked RVs. Walk northwest along this road until you come to the California Riding and Hiking Trail (see page 38) at 5.25 miles. Note that you'll see two markers here. Go left (west) onto the narrow, single-track trail.

At 6.3 miles, the route begins descending toward Box Canyon. You'll spot the historic marker alongside S2 on your right. The plaque tells of the Mormon Battalion using hand tools to gouge out the first road into Southern California. The route continues on mostly level ground alongside S2 all the way back to the parking turnout.

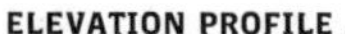

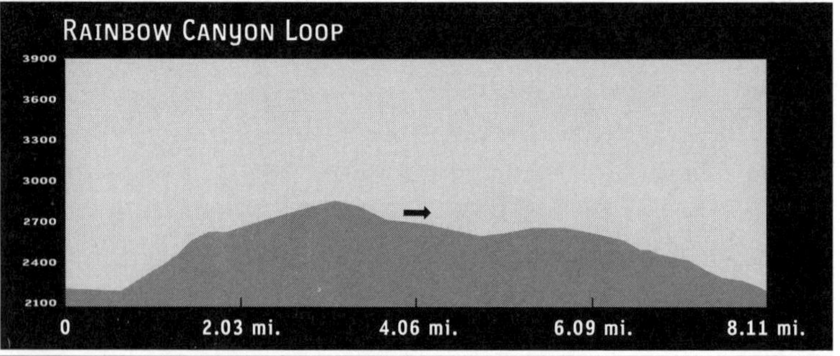

Directions: Take CA 78 to S2 and go south, then continue just over 9 miles to a wide turnout on the east side of the highway, south of mile marker 27, and park.

GPS Coordinates	16 RAINBOW CANYON LOOP
UTM Zone (WGS84)	11S
Easting	550780
Northing	3652244
Latitude–Longitude	N 33° 0' 26.8049"
	W 116° 27' 22.9140"

17 Oriflamme Canyon

SCENERY: ★★★★★
DIFFICULTY: ★★★★
TRAIL CONDITION: ★★
SOLITUDE: ★★★★
CHILDREN: ★

DISTANCE: *5–10 miles round trip*
HIKING TIME: *2.5–6 hours*
OUTSTANDING FEATURES: *Wide variety of desert and riparian vegetation, a flowing seasonal creek with sparkling pools, waterfalls, and the accompanying serene sounds*

Beginning in Blair Valley at an elevation of around 2,300 feet and climbing to around 3,200 feet, this out-and-back hike takes you through a vegetation-rich ecotone between low and high desert. In wet years or after sufficient rainfall, the seasonal creek, Vallecito Wash, will be running. The last 1.4-mile section (perhaps your four-wheel-drive starting point; see option below) transports you into a tangle of riparian wilderness that will make you forget you're in the desert. The rugged terrain climbs through creek-fed cottonwoods, willows, and sycamore trees, leading past several small waterfalls to the sloshing endpoint: falls that tumble approximately 15 feet from the craggy rock face into the gurgling stream below.

OPTION: *With a four-wheel drive, you can drive the first 3 miles along a dirt road and park above a stream to pick up the last 1.4 miles of the trail. The option shaves the hike to 2.8 round-trip miles along the wash (the toughest, and perhaps the most rewarding portion of the trail). This would also be a good place to camp, remembering the park rules not to bed down too close to the water sources, as it might disturb wildlife.*

Begin walking southwest along the dirt Oriflamme Canyon Road. After a short distance, turn right, heading northwest along the fairly flat road. If you were to continue southwest, a locked private gate at about 0.25 miles would block your progress. This flat, rather uneventful road, save the occasional darting cottontail or jackrabbit, allows for a brisk aerobic workout. The terrain is spotted abundantly with creosote bushes, recognizable by their small, dark-green leaves,

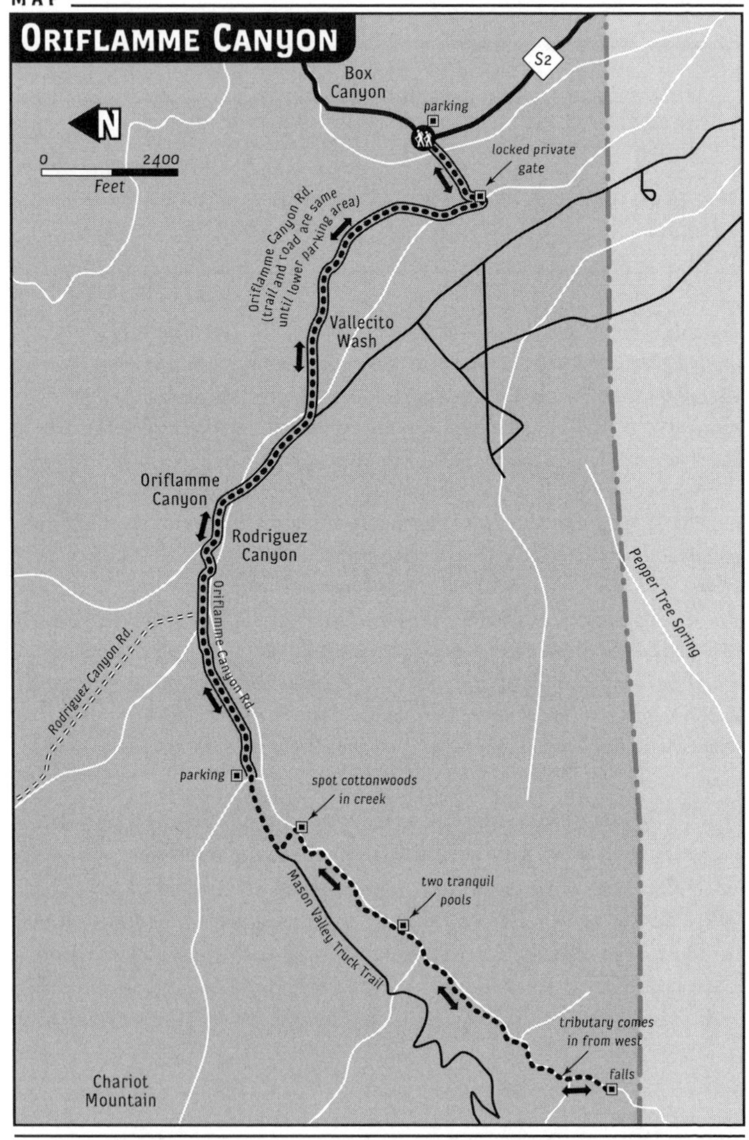
Oriflamme Canyon
N
0
2400
Feet
Box Canyon
S2
parking
locked private gate
Oriflamme Canyon Rd. (trail and road are same until lower parking area)
Vallecito Wash
Oriflamme Canyon
Rodriguez Canyon
Rodriguez Canyon Rd.
Oriflamme Canyon Rd.
Pepper Tree Spring
parking
spot cottonwoods in creek
Mason Valley Truck Trail
two tranquil pools
tributary comes in from west
falls
Chariot Mountain

yellow flowers with sparse, separate petals, and pea-sized fruits covered in white fuzz. Note the uniform space that exists between the plants, caused by a germination-inhibitor that is secreted by the roots and prevents new seedlings from becoming established within the plant's circular root zone. This is one of the creosote bush's defenses against drought.

After approximately 1.8 miles, reach a fork where Rodriguez Canyon Road (also dirt) comes in on the right. Take the left fork, marked "Oriflamme Canyon," and continue as the road curves more southwest again for about another mile. To your left, you'll spot cottonwood trees in the creek bed and eventually reach a short dirt road that leads southeast to the creek itself (from Oriflamme Canyon Road, which continues). Park here if you've brought the four-wheel drive. This point is the location of a historic mining camp. The gold-producing Oriflamme Mine was probably named for miners who arrived in San Diego in 1870 on a steamship named *Oriflamme.*

Turn right at the canyon bottom, following the water (if present) or creek bed upstream (southwest). Occasionally stoop under tangles of low sycamore branches and push through limber willow trees as

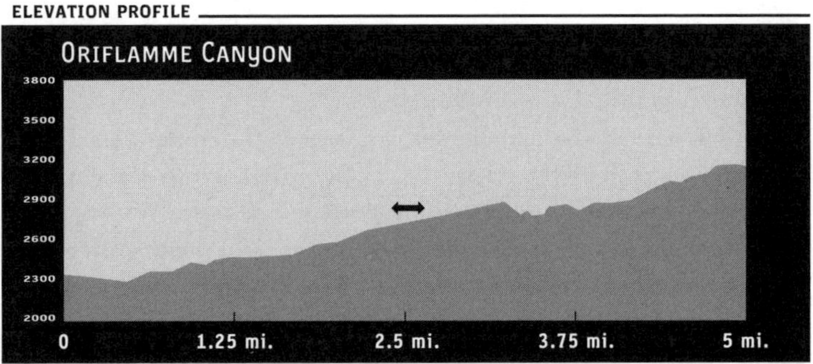

you slowly tread along. Don't follow other hikers too closely—the whiplike branches may snap back and slap you. When the creek is running, the soft gurgle adds a pleasing backdrop to this beautiful, shaded route. This is prime picnicking land, particularly in fall when the hand-shaped sycamore leaves turn a vibrant orange-gold and create a soft blanket of groundcover. The leaf cover is deep in spots, sometimes causing unexpected sinking as you step. Also, as is warned in all desert areas, be extra cautious of rattlesnakes in warm weather.

Pick your way along on either side of the creek, crossing as needed to make progress and keep your feet dry. There are plenty of small boulders and flattish rocks on which to step. After about 0.5 miles, the creek reaches a tranquil spot where two decent-sized pools (approximate areas of 60 and 200 square feet) are fed by a series of short falls—smaller sisters to that at the hike's climax. For those who don't want to thread their way through thickening vegetation, this is a sensible, rewarding turnaround point. But for those who love solitude and don't mind a slow, rough trek through thick vegetation into quiet wilderness, this spot only whets the appetite for nature's treasures to come.

To move ahead, you'll need to climb around the craggy boulders to the right, accessing a narrow, easy trail that will lead you away from, then back down to, the creek. This single-track trail is actually the remnants of a cow path, which will intermittently appear and disappear in varying degrees of ease for the rest of this hike. Oriflamme Canyon was once a cattle-running route and stretches from here into the Laguna Mountains.

When the easy cow path delivers you back to the creek, cross it, then find the path on the other side. The canyon narrows at times, requiring you to cross and recross the creek several times, finding threads of decent path among dense thickets of spiny desert apricot, bushy lemonade berry, mallow plants with their cupped, coral flowers, red-bloomed chuparosa, willows, and even a few spindly primrose bushes. In the fall and early winter, when leaves are dry and plants drop their seeds, you'll develop a healthy respect for the cocklebur plant. Its narrow, inch-long burs grab and hold onto socks, shoes, pants, packs, and sleeves. The burs have an uncanny way of latching onto shoelaces, causing even double-tied knots to loosen. Fuzzy fabrics like fleece will literally be coated with the burs in a matter of minutes—much as a cow's hide might have been as it passed through on this old cattle route.

Continue along the creek. In some areas, it's easiest to tightly hug the stream, enjoying its algae-bearded stones, tiny eddies, and trickling Zen spots. Close to a mile past the small falls with their tranquil pair of pools, you'll reach a tributary coming in from the right (west). Approximately 0.1 mile past this point, as the trail climbs along above the right side of the creek, spot the 15-foot falls cascading into the creek below.

On the way out, gravity aids your travel back down the creek bed as you move with ease, flowing like water over stones and branches. Be careful, though, because a misstep can mean a tumble. If you prefer a clearer route, when you reach the point where you accessed the easy cow path above the set of tranquil pools, continue along this path (moving northwest) to a point on the dirt road just a short walk from where you accessed the creek (and/or perhaps left your four-wheel drive). Retrace your steps along Oriflamme Canyon Road back to the parking site (trailhead) along County Route S2.

Directions: Take CA 78 to County Route S2 and turn south, then continue approximately 9 miles to Oriflamme Canyon Road (a dirt road on the right between mile markers 26 and 27). Pull off and park in one of the small turnouts (see shorter option above for four-wheel-drive vehicles).

GPS Coordinates	17 ORIFLAMME CANYON
UTM Zone (WGS84)	11S
Easting	550780
Northing	3652244
Latitude–Longitude	N 33° 0' 26.8049"
	W 116° 27' 22.9140"

18 The Mortreros

SCENERY: ☆☆☆
DIFFICULTY: ☆
TRAIL CONDITION: ☆☆☆☆☆
SOLITUDE: ☆☆
CHILDREN: ☆☆☆☆☆

DISTANCE: *0.6 miles round trip*
HIKING TIME: *0.5–1 hour*
OUTSTANDING FEATURES: *Huge boulder groupings with Native American mortreros; possible wildlife including quail, coyotes, and doves*

This nearly flat, easy trail leads to the historic site of a Kumeyaay village where the rocks hold evidence of Indian family life.

The short, easy trail slopes gradually upward, but with only 60 feet gained over the 0.25 miles out, the climb will hardly be noticed. During the walk, listen for the calls of quail, watch for jackrabbits, and enjoy the vast space of the sky overhead. Native Americans who lived here in the milder months of September to May beginning more than 1,000 years ago would have been alert to these same sounds of nature.

Just a few steps onto this wide, sandy trail lead you to huge boulder groupings, which upon close inspection reveal mortreros—the bowl-like pits formed in the rocks where Native Americans ground mesquite beans into meal. Mixed with water, the mesquite-bean meal became a thick, edible mush. The Kumeyaay also formed cakes from the mush, which they dried for later eating, perhaps during journeys into surrounding mountains to collect piñon nuts—another nutrient-rich food staple. The Indians utilized all parts of their food sources, using mesquite from root to leaves. Spring blooms were brewed into a tea or roasted and eaten. Tea from mesquite leaves helped remedy diarrhea, leaves and twigs offered disinfectant properties for cuts and scrapes, while the pods offered a conjunctivitis cure.

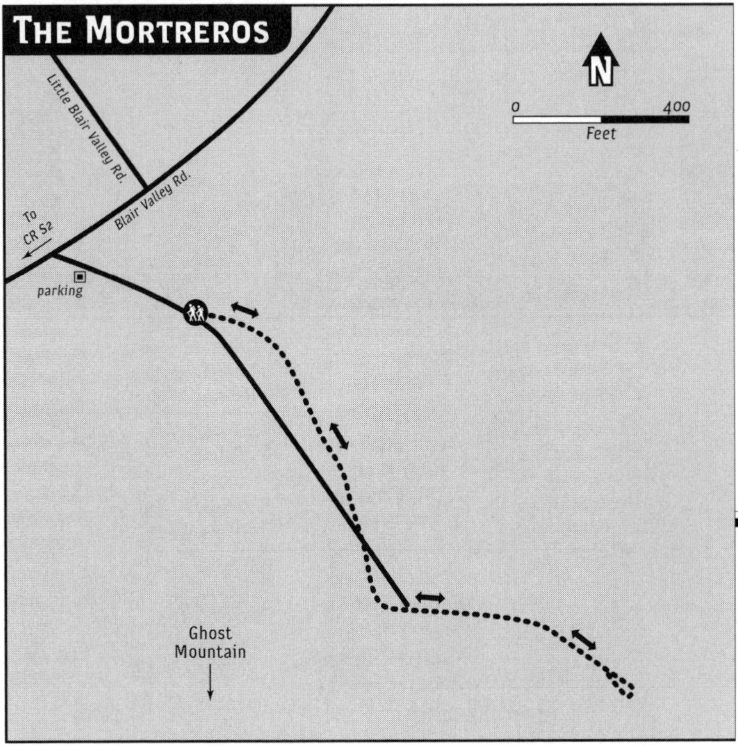

MAP

The Mortreros

N
0 400
Feet
Little Blair Valley Rd.
Blair Valley Rd.
To CR S2
parking
Ghost Mountain

As you ponder what it might have been like to live in this rocky village, you may be tempted to imitate the actions of ancient peoples by kneeling atop one of the wide boulders and using a small smooth rock to grind imaginary seeds in one of the many depressions. Resist the urge, though—this is an archaeological site, and disturbing it is against the law.

ELEVATION PROFILE

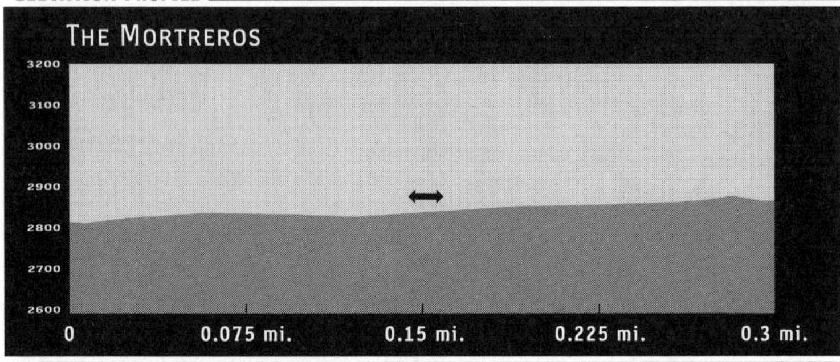

Directions: Where Highway 78 meets County Route S2 (the Great Overland Route of 1849), head south on S2 for 6.4 miles to Blair Valley Road. Turn left onto this flat, dirt road suitable for most vehicles. After approximately 3.5 miles, park in the pullout on the right, marked "Mortreros."

GPS Coordinates	18 THE MORTREROS
UTM Zone (WGS84)	11S
Easting	558076
Northing	3652440
Latitude–Longitude	N 33° 0' 31.8779"
	W 116° 22' 41.7026"

19 Pictograph Trail

SCENERY: ☆☆☆
DIFFICULTY: ☆
TRAIL CONDITION: ☆☆☆☆☆
SOLITUDE: ☆☆
CHILDREN: ☆☆☆☆

DISTANCE: *2.8 miles round trip*
HIKING TIME: *0.5–1 hour*
OUTSTANDING FEATURES: *Sandy wash, Native American rock art, and a valley view*

This flat, easy trail travels straight over sandy wash and passes next to a display of native Indian rock art (pictographs). The path then leads to a sudden drop-off overlook into the Vallecitos Valley. The up close view of the rock art symbols at 0.8 miles and the easy hiking make this a good choice for school-age children, but be careful if you hike the remaining 0.6 miles to the overlook. The drop-off is abrupt, so don't let children run ahead.

The easy trail slopes gradually upward, stretching 0.8 miles to a huge boulder decorated with rock art that features symbols from the ancient Kumeyaay Indian residents of the valley. The boulder is right next to the path, making the art's preserved nature that much more remarkable. Researchers don't know for sure what the 200- to 300-year-old symbols represent, but the diamond-chain motifs are typical of other Indian artifacts. This historic rock art is rendered with paints made from ground minerals that endure constant natural erosion from the elements (wind, sun, rain). Please help preserve them for the enjoyment of future visitors. Don't touch or deface the pictographs, which are protected by law. Instead, bring your camera and consider what the symbols might have meant to the men and women who created them.

The sandy trail grows wider, the soft ground imprinted with the tracks of local wildlife such as jackrabbits, quail, and coyotes. Fairly fresh mountain-lion tracks were present on my last visit during the

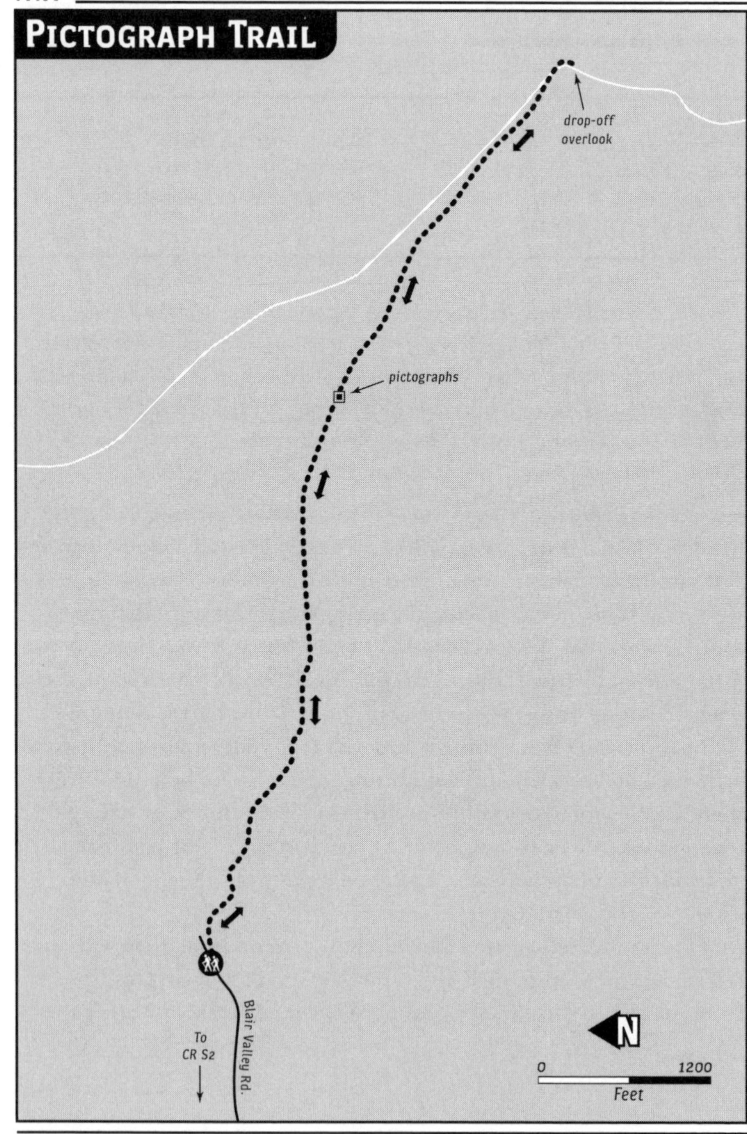
PICTOGRAPH TRAIL
drop-off
overlook
pictographs
Blair Valley Rd.
To
CR S2
N
0
1200
Feet

winter months. The sandy wash continues another 0.5 miles toward a ridgeline that appears to block the path. Several hundred yards from the trail's end, though, a cleft appears, allowing entrance into a great stone hallway of sorts. The thick rock walls rise on either side of the path, ushering you through. Watch your step—the path ends abruptly on an unshielded precipice. Ever wary of the 100- to 200-foot drop-off, admire the view over the Vallecitos Valley before retracing your steps to the trailhead.

ELEVATION PROFILE

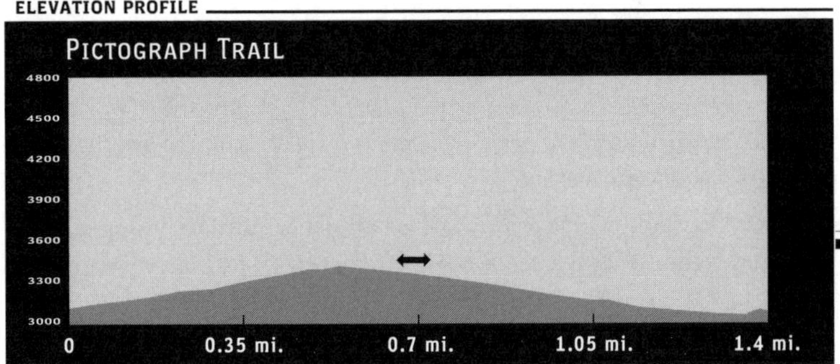

Directions: Where CA 78 meets County Route S2 (the Great Overland Route of 1849), head south on S2 for 6.4 miles to Blair Valley Road. Turn left onto this flat, dirt road suitable for most vehicles. After approximately 3.5 miles, a fork joins the road. Follow the sign leading to the Pictograph Trail (left). After another 1.5 miles, the road ends in a large parking turnout. The trailhead sign is on the right.

GPS Coordinates	**19 PICTOGRAPH TRAIL**
UTM Zone (WGS84)	**11S**
Easting	**559802**
Northing	**3653644**
Latitude–Longitude	**N 33° 1' 10.6309"**
	W 116° 21' 34.9147"

20 Ghost Mountain

SCENERY: ★★★★
DIFFICULTY: ★★★
TRAIL CONDITION: ★★★★
SOLITUDE: ★★
CHILDREN: ★★★
DISTANCE: *1.4 miles round trip*
HIKING TIME: *1 hour*
OUTSTANDING FEATURES: *A climbing path to the home site of the South family, who lived at the top of this mountain, perhaps the proverbial "top of the world" to this creative, colorful couple and their children.*

The history evident on this immediately climbing trail makes the hike a wonder from the first step. The Souths, a family who lived on Ghost Mountain in the 1930s and 1940s, carefully placed rocks along the route that still provide good footing. The quiet mountaintop, with its ruins of the family's rural lifestyle, offers a pretty view and sparks imaginings about how they lived.

The path begins at the base of Ghost Mountain and quickly becomes steep. A level stretch begins after just 0.4 miles, allowing a breather as a southerly view of the Vallecitos Valley, backed by the Sawtooth Mountains, appears beyond the rocky trail. The trail continues northeast, beginning to climb steeply in spots that make you appreciate the efforts of the family who once lived here. Steps have been whittled into existing exposed rock in some areas, while stones have been lodged in place for easier footing in others.

After a short distance, the trail again levels. Easy ground leads to the dilapidated remains of the cabin home of painter-writer Marshall South; his wife, Tanya; and their three children. They called the cabin "Yaquitepec," a combination of two Indian words that refer to the Souths' quest for freedom on this desert hill. An old water cistern is nearby, as well as a shallow pool and other artifacts from their rainwater collection efforts. The trail continues for approximately another 0.1 mile, ending at an outcropping of boulders overlooking the valley below.

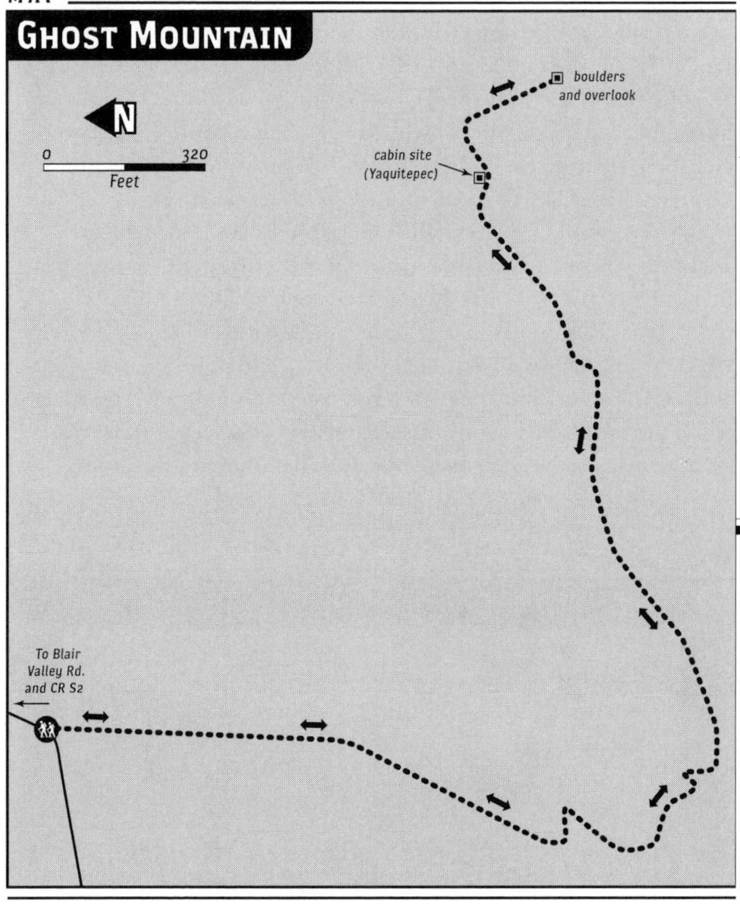
GHOST MOUNTAIN
N
0
320
Feet
boulders
and overlook
cabin site
(Yaquitepec)
To Blair
Valley Rd.
and CR S2

Give yourself time to sit and ponder how it must have been to live virtually cut off from civilization other than your immediate family. (And take care to note that this is a historic site, which should be enjoyed but not disturbed.) The Souths called Ghost Mountain home for 16 years, during which Marshall South penned regular articles about their desert lifestyle for *Desert Magazine*. The couple then divorced. Tanya, a poet, took their three children and reentered San Diego civilization, while Marshall moved to Julian. *San Diego Union-Tribune* newspaper articles and historical accounts speculate about how happy the family really was during their time on Ghost Mountain.

Other than the remnants of the South family's life and a lovely view, the hike offers an aerobic workout up and down the steep path. On my last visit, I met an active 89-year-old woman treading along the trail, which climbs approximately 400 feet in quick succession, proving that hiking may indeed be the fountain of youth.

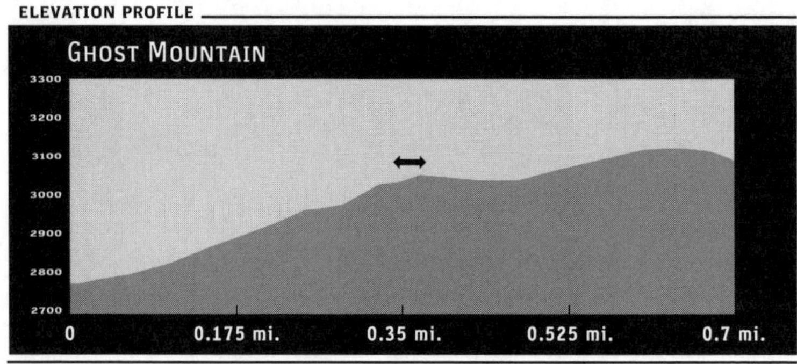

Directions: Where CA 78 meets County Route S2 (the Great Overland Route of 1849), head south on S2 for 6.4 miles to Blair Valley Road. Turn left onto this flat, dirt road suitable for most vehicles and follow the signs (bearing right) to Ghost Mountain, about 2.4 miles. Parking turnouts are next to the trailhead sign on the left.

GPS Coordinates	20 GHOST MOUNTAIN
UTM Zone (WGS84)	11S
Easting	557008
Northing	3651825
Latitude–Longitude	N 33° 0' 12.0996"
	W 116° 23' 23.0047"

area five

BOW WILLOW AND MOUNTAIN PALM SPRINGS

5

Many
consider
the
desert
dry
and desolate
but
secret oases
cool
waterfalls
interesting
animals
and
a wide
array of
adaptive
vegetation
wait
quietly
to refresh
adventurous
souls

AREA 5: Bow Willow and Mountain Palm Springs

Introduction

The Bow Willow and Mountain Palm Springs campgrounds lie adjacent to one another along County Route S2 in the southern part of the Anza-Borrego Desert State Park. Located south of the Tierra Blanca Mountains and nestled amid arid surrounding desert, both campgrounds offer good base points for nearby hikes. A few of the possibilities are described here, allowing a glimpse at palm oases and historical points of interest that will whet the appetite for further desert exploration.

The Mountain Palm Springs Loop delivers you into sandy washes with underground springs that feed palm groves that, in turn, sustain the wildlife. Indian Valley (accessed via the Indian Gorge Trail, which is part of the loop) was once home to the Kumeyaay Indians, who would have used Indian Gorge as a footpath to the fan palms. The trees' fruit was ground into flour or soaked to concoct a sweet drink, while the fibrous leaves were used for shelter and clothes. Elephant trees, which are more fully described in the Alma Wash and Elephant Tree Nature Trail write-ups, cling to the walls of Torote Canyon and grow above the Southwest Grove. They are abundant in Torote Bowl (southwest of Mountain Palm Springs and northeast of the Bow Willow Campground).

The Bow Willow–Rockhouse Canyon Loop takes you through boulder-studded gorges, to a historic cattleman's shack made of stone, and through a sandy wash where water sometimes flows in abundance.

Camping at Mountain Palm Springs means little more than flat turnout areas, while Bow Willow is a bit more developed, with picnic benches and shaded areas. While both are good starting points for day hikes, backpacking out for overnight tent stays might be fun. Exploring farther into the surrounding mountains, up the sandy washes, or into Bow Willow Canyon, Torote Canyon, or Indian Valley make good options for remote desert camping. Indian Valley can be accessed via Indian Gorge Road (just north of Mountain Palm Springs), which is a dirt route that requires a four-wheel drive. The valley has a south and north fork with palms. The south fork features some Indian mortreros and an old shelter cave.

21 Bow Willow–Rockhouse Canyon Loop

Scenery: ☆☆☆
Difficulty: ☆☆☆
Trail Condition: ☆☆☆
Solitude: ☆☆☆☆
Children: ☆☆

Distance: *8.5 miles round trip*
Hiking Time: *4.5–5 hours*
Outstanding Features: *Sandy wash, seasonal water, and a historic cattleman's rock shelter*

This trail takes you from the semiprimitive setting of the Bow Willow Campground south into Rockhouse Canyon to glimpse Depression-era relics. You'll travel from people to solitude and see unusual rock formations as well as a variety of desert vegetation. Brief climbs and descents over varying terrain are interspersed with long, flat treks across sandy washes and open desert. After spring rains, refreshing water gushes through Bow Willow Valley.

From the dirt parking areas at the end of the Bow Willow Campground, head northeast, veering almost immediately left (west) into the wide wash of Bow Willow Valley. After about 0.5 miles on flat, sandy terrain, you'll turn left again, heading into a narrow gorge filled with sweet-smelling desert lilac and red-bloomed chuparosa bushes. After about 0.2 miles, you'll have to step over some smaller boulders, dodging the grasp of acacia catclaw and passing a single fan palm. The boulders' sizes and occurrence increase as you move ahead, but the rocks aren't difficult to work around or over as the path gradually begins to gain elevation. Climb for less than 0.5 miles, then reach flat wash and continue moving southwest.

At 1.6 miles from the trailhead, or 0.6 miles up-wash, you'll reach a yellow-topped pole marker. Veer to the right here and continue through an area populated by interesting boulder formations and cholla for another 0.5 miles or so. You'll reach a natural rock "wall" with rock ducks perched atop. Climb over the rocks to the other side. Look for a dilapidated yellow marker just ahead and to the left; beyond this stands a rock grouping that forms a tunnel and a natural

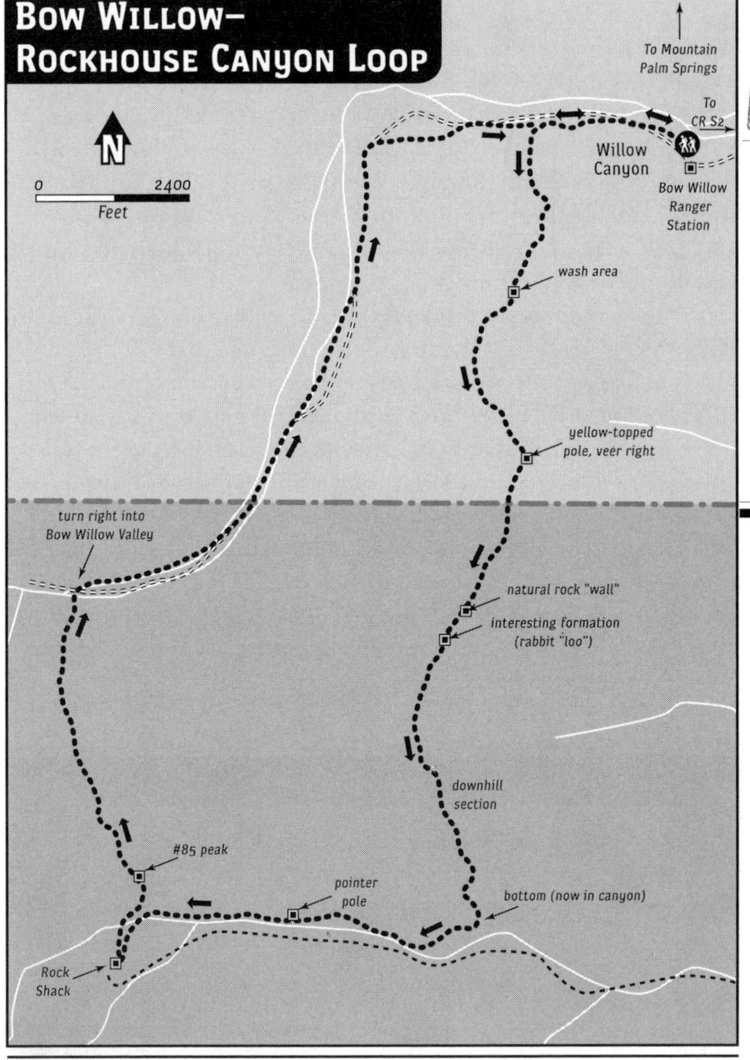
Bow Willow–
Rockhouse Canyon Loop
N
0
2400
Feet
To Mountain
Palm Springs
To
CR S2
Willow
Canyon
Bow Willow
Ranger
Station
wash area
yellow-topped
pole, veer right
turn right into
Bow Willow Valley
natural rock "wall"
interesting formation
(rabbit "loo")
downhill
section
#85 peak
pointer
pole
bottom (now in canyon)
Rock
Shack

courtyard—probably called "the loo" by rabbits, if what's inside is an indication. From there, the trail is sometimes not so easily identified. Watch for foot-tracks on a route arcing gradually left, and the ever-present rock ducks left by other hikers to guide you.

Approximately 0.25 miles ahead from the "loo," you'll enter a rocky downhill divide (still marked by ducks). Be careful of desert apricot, with its narrow branches ending in many pointy spines. At first, this is an easy downhill stroll on evident trail. Boulders soon encroach, though, requiring climbs up and over and perhaps sitting and sliding down the front.

At the bottom of the divide, turn right, walking west on flat terrain thick with prickly cholla. Stay toward the north side of the valley. The idea is to locate a yellow-topped marker pole at 0.5 miles from the turn at the bottom of the divide, then continue on for another 0.5 miles to the second marker. At this point, look for the rockhouse, which rests against the south wall of the canyon and is difficult to spot at first. The easiest way to see the shelter, which tends to blend into the surroundings, is to first look across the canyon and find the metal piping that runs down the south canyon wall. Then locate the rockhouse, which is tucked at the base of the hill, just west of the piping. Once you see it, head directly across (about 0.25 miles) to experience its relic charm.

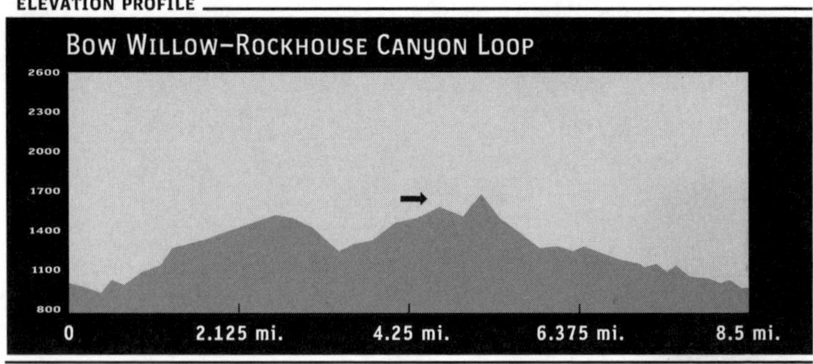

With a rusty metal roof and piled-rock walls, the small stone shelter is supported by old beams and still holds some metal bedsprings. In one corner you can see the remnants of a fireplace, a humble hearth where a work-weary cattleman may have warmed water or grub. Historical information states that the cabin was built in 1933. The piping hails from a seasonal spring located a short distance up the hill.

From the rockhouse, the historic highlight of this trek, head back across the canyon to the marker pole, and move west to make your way over the ridge. The route is steep but is only 0.25 miles to the peak and won't require handholds. Follow the steep and rather slippery zigzag path down the other side, back into Bow Willow Valley. In wetter years, particularly after spring rains, you may find water gushing through the valley. Linger awhile streamside if you like. From here it's about 3 easy, flat miles east back to the trailhead. In winter, look for clumps of mistletoe growing in bushes and trees, and listen for the soft, single-note call of the phainopepla, which resembles a black cardinal. You may spot the bird's crested head as it perches for a few moments, resting between its flitting travels to feast upon mistletoe berries.

Directions: Where CA 78 meets County Route S2 (the Great Overland Route of 1849), head south for 31.2 miles. En route, you'll see the sign marking your entrance into Anza-Borrego Desert State Park at approximately 4.4 miles. After 21 miles, veer left to continue on S2. A sign marks the Bow Willow Campground at 31.2 miles. Turn right, driving 1.7 miles on this flat, dirt road to the end of the campground, where day-use parking is marked by cut telephone poles lying on their sides.

GPS Coordinates	21 BOW WILLOW–ROCKHOUSE CANYON LOOP
UTM Zone (WGS84)	11S
Easting	572371
Northing	3634168
Latitude–Longitude	N 32° 50' 35.4731" W 116° 13' 35.9563"

22 Mountain Palm Springs Loop

SCENERY: ☆☆☆
DIFFICULTY: ☆☆☆
TRAIL CONDITION: ☆☆☆
SOLITUDE: ☆☆☆
CHILDREN: ☆☆

DISTANCE: *7.4 miles round trip*
HIKING TIME: *0.5–6 hours*
OUTSTANDING FEATURES: *Palm oases, sandy wash, seasonal water, and sweeping views of the desert*

Six palm groves of varying sizes, two within quick access to the trailhead (which itself is easily reached from County Route S2) make Mountain Palm Springs a visitor favorite. Primitive camping here, and close proximity to more developed Bow Willow Campground just over the hill, also contribute to its popularity. It's a busy location and you're likely to see others, especially at the large Southwest Grove, which provides access to 1.5 miles of flat trail from the parking area.

OPTIONS: *Overnight stays—primitive camping at Mountain Palm Springs itself or at the Bow Willow Campground (which can be accessed via the Torote Bowl Trail from Southwest Grove). As alternatives to the overview loop route described in detail below, shorter round-trip day hike choices include a northwest trek to and from Mary's Grove (0.8 miles), a southwesterly walk to and from the Southwest Grove (3 miles), and side trails to explore the Indian Gorge trail and Torote Canyon (see notations in the description). The maximum mileage of 7.8 includes Indian Gorge and Torote Canyon in this loop.*

For a look at all six area palm groves, this loop route begins by heading northwest on a flat sandy wash toward the only palms visible from the parking trailhead (Mary's Grove). This easy stroll to shady Mary's Grove makes a wonderful out-and-back option, perhaps as a pleasant break on a long Sunday drive. Seasonal above-ground water flow makes an orchestra of trickling water a possibility. Abundant underground water supports the oases. At about 0.33 miles, you'll encounter a few boulders that are easily stepped over before you reach the outskirts of this first oasis at 0.4 miles. Explore

3/24/08 Part way at night. Came back in dark w/ headlamps. Encounter w/ owl (burrowing?) Beautiful area, great trail

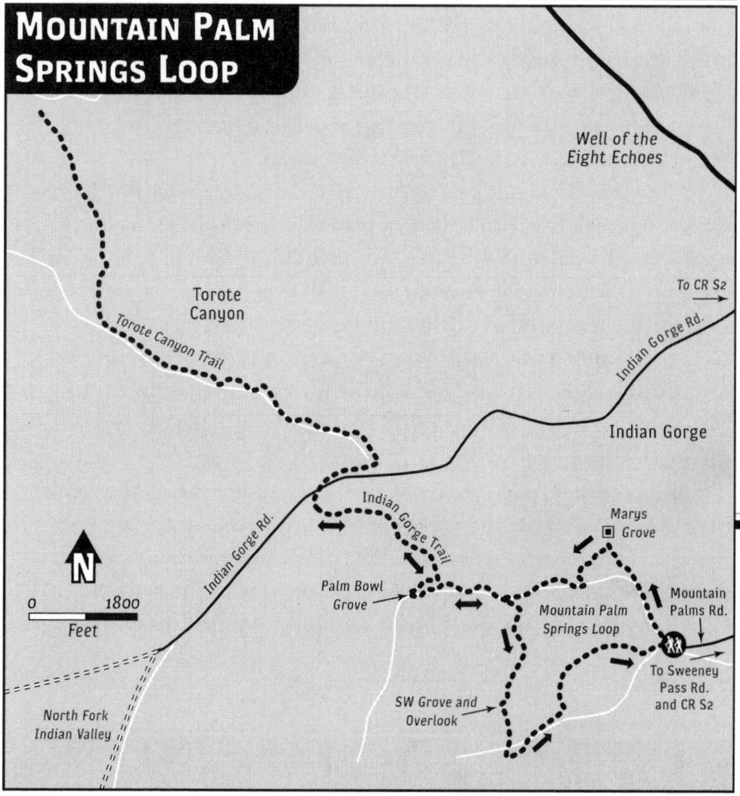

Mountain Palm Springs Loop

Well of the Eight Echoes
Torote Canyon
Torote Canyon Trail
To CR S2
Indian Gorge Rd.
Indian Gorge
Indian Gorge Trail
Marys Grove
N
0 1800 Feet
Palm Bowl Grove
Mountain Palm Springs Loop
Mountain Palms Rd.
To Sweeney Pass Rd. and CR S2
SW Grove and Overlook
North Fork Indian Valley

a little farther along the line of trees in Mary's Grove, pausing for a while if you wish.

To connect to the loop, turn left almost immediately upon reaching Mary's Grove (thought to be named for an area store owner) and enter a narrow gorge that hosts a small cluster of palms.

Continue along on either side of the palms, up the short gorge to the top of the ridge. From here, find the steep path down into the canyon, careful not to slip on the crumbly soil as you descend. Head right, moving west for about 0.2 miles, and you'll reach tiny North Grove, which looks like a few straggler palms compared to larger Surprise Canyon Grove already visible ahead.

Continue west and pass by Surprise Canyon Grove, but for the return trip, take note of a narrow trail that begins here, heading up the south side of the canyon. It's difficult to spot at first, so find the path by looking for rock ducks left by others to mark the route. Leave it for now, and continue up the canyon toward Palm Bowl Grove, about 0.33 miles ahead. This section is thickly overgrown with thorny acacia catclaw. Staying to the left (north) side of the canyon offers the best route, with open paths moving easily through the vicious bushes.

In the winter, you'll hear the one-note call of the phainopepla here, and possibly see the dark, crested bird flittering among the catclaw. Squirrels scamper about the rocky canyon sides. On my last visit, I startled a large owl that had captured one of the rodents. Clutching its prey, the great bird flew silently to the tops of the palms.

ELEVATION PROFILE

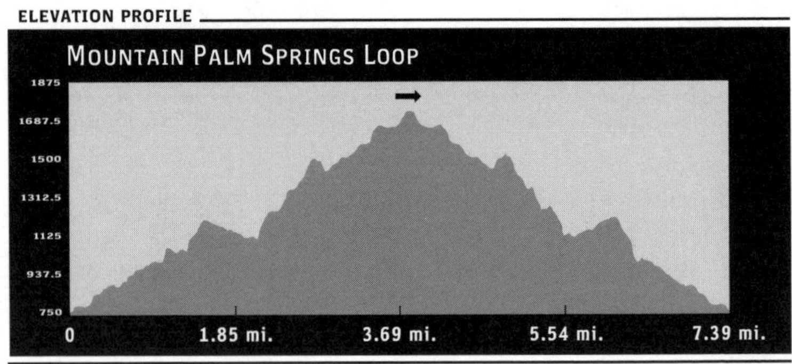

Spend a little time exploring the shady amphitheater delights of peaceful Palm Bowl Grove. Listen for the trickling, echoing sound of ripe berries falling from the treetops, perhaps dislodged by hungry birds. Doves and orioles, as well as coyotes, frequent the cool, food-abundant area.

Next, retrace your steps eastward. To extend the hike outside of Mountain Palm Springs for an introduction to the surrounding area, look for the Indian Gorge Trail, which heads up the north side of the canyon just east of Palm Bowl Grove. Unless you're searching, you're not likely to see this trail at all. Careful examination will probably reveal some rock ducks arranged near the base. At one time, the bare stem of a palm frond stood up in the sand to mark the path. Hikers often try to help each other. You may or may not find a definitive marker.

The Indian Gorge Trail itself climbs steeply for about 0.1 mile, then flattens and gradually descends into Indian Valley. The whole stretch of easy trail is 0.5 miles, adding a round-trip mile to the loop. If you have the time and inclination to add another 3.6 miles of hiking, go the short distance across the valley to Indian Gorge Road (dirt), turn right and walk approximately 0.2 miles to the opening of Torote Canyon (see page 133), and hike its 1.6 miles each way before connecting back with the Indian Gorge Trail and continuing on the Mountain Palm Springs loop.

Back at the base of the Indian Gorge Trail, near Palm Bowl Grove, go left (east), and retrace your steps to Surprise Canyon Grove. Find the trail you located on your first pass, leading up the canyon wall. The narrow trail begins a southwesterly track but quickly veers southeast, steeply climbing on the edge of the canyon wall up to the ridge, then veering southwest (away from the edge) again. The rocky trail through dry landscape is fairly easy to follow for about 0.5 miles; then the Southwest Grove appears suddenly down below. From this tranquil vantage point, the wind sounds like ocean waves as it rustles through the palm leaves.

A narrow, steep trail leads down into the oasis. Be sure to look for the elephant trees as you descend. A large one clings to the canyon wall alongside the descending trail. For a close-up look at these interesting trees with red inner flesh and twisting trunks, consider hiking the Torote Bowl trail. You can access it at the north side of the Southwest Grove. There, a sign marks the trail, which heads upward for 0.5 miles to a grove of the large trees. The Torote Bowl trail connects to another path, descending approximately 1 mile into the Bow Willow Campground.

Once you finish your tour of these desert oases that draw wildlife from the arid surroundings, take the trail from the Southwest Grove leading northeast. It's approximately 1.5 miles of easy strolling—your feet may get wet in seasonal water flow—to your car. Along the way, you'll pass through Pygmy Grove, recognized by its smaller palms.

Directions: Where Highway 78 meets County Route S2 (the Great Overland Route of 1849), turn right and head south on S2 for 29.4 miles. En route, you'll see the sign marking your entrance into Anza-Borrego Desert State Park at approximately 4.4 miles. After 21 miles, veer left to continue on S2. A sign marks Mountain Palm Springs at 29.4 miles. Turn right, driving 0.5 miles on the smooth dirt road, past primitive camping turnouts, to parking areas on the right and left.

GPS Coordinates	22 MOUNTAIN PALM SPRINGS LOOP
UTM Zone (WGS84)	11S
Easting	573096
Northing	3636325
Latitude–Longitude	N 32° 51' 45.3389" W 116° 13' 7.4764"

23 Torote Canyon

Scenery: ★★★	Distance: *3.2 miles round trip*
Difficulty: ★★★	Hiking Time: *2–3 hours*
Trail Condition: ★★★	Outstanding Features: *Sandy wash, columnar barrel cactus, smoke trees, jackrabbits, quail, and quiet*
Solitude: ★★★★	
Children: ★★	

A few steps into the canyon on this relatively short hike bring peace, quiet, and a sense of distance from the world. In the wide, sandy wash of Torote Canyon, walk along with an ease that requires little attention to your steps—making this an excellent day hike for solitude lost in thought, or for sharing uninterrupted conversation with a companion. A narrower offshoot gorge requires more careful footing, delivering you to a wide, rocky bowl—either a turnaround point or the climbing gateway into surrounding desert.

You'll see a dilapidated marker at the trailhead (no writing remains on its face). Park here, and walk northwest into the narrow canyon mouth. Almost immediately, you'll see elephant trees—also known as torote—clinging to the canyon walls. *Torote* is Spanish for "to twist," which appropriately describes the tree's twisting branches. After approximately 0.5 miles, the chasm widens, the trees disappear, and desert lavender scents the air. As you move along, your footsteps sink into the soft, sandy wash—perhaps startling jackrabbits from beneath the fragrant brush. Tumbled rock lines the route, gilded with dark desert varnish on the north side.

At a little more than a mile, the route forks, and you'll veer to the right into a narrower side gorge. The path climbs a little but remains a fairly easygoing trek and flattens again after a short ascent. Continue north toward the now-visible end of the canyon, moving past some good-sized columnar barrel cactus—abloom in spring—growing beside one another like field goals along the path.

MAP

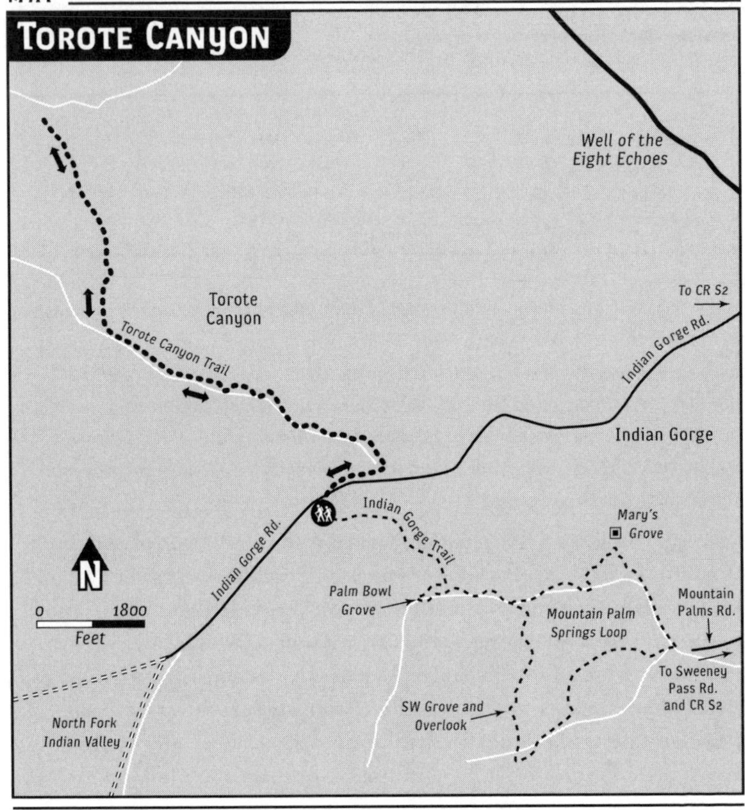

The path ends in a bowl of sorts that's lined with various-sized boulders and spiny cholla cactus. There are stretches of rocky, packed sand in between. If you want to, you can climb out of the bowl, traveling without too much difficulty a few more miles across rock-studded terrain into the Canebrake area. Scrambling a few yards up the rocks for a perching spot is usually enough for me. The view down canyon is a pretty reward.

This is a good place to sit and eat lunch, reflect, and contemplate the stark beauty of the desert. Take a few moments to listen to the breeze, let the sun's warmth caress your skin, and enjoy the vast blue sky. You may see busy hummingbirds, meandering quail, or grazing jackrabbits that frequent Torote Canyon.

ELEVATION PROFILE

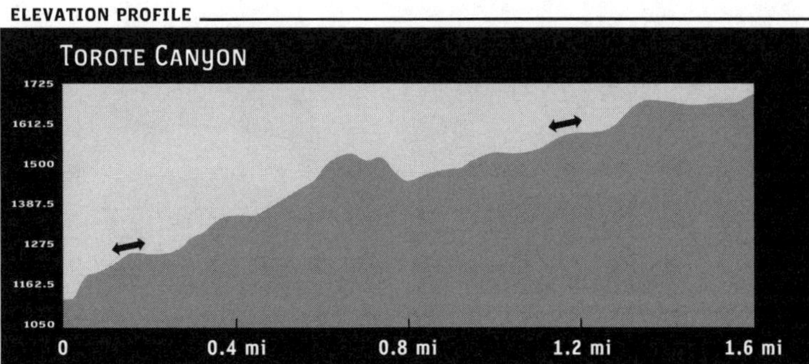

Directions: Where CA 78 meets County Route S2 (the Great Overland Route of 1849), head south on S2 for 28 miles. En route, you'll see the sign marking your entrance into Anza-Borrego Desert State Park at approximately 4.4 miles. After 21 miles, veer left to continue on S2. A sign marks Indian Gorge at approximately 28 miles. Turn right, driving 1.8 miles to the Torote Canyon trailhead on the right.

GPS Coordinates	23 TOROTE CANYON
UTM Zone (WGS84)	11S
Easting	571576
Northing	3637197
Latitude–Longitude	N 32° 52' 14.0299"
	W 116° 14' 5.7057"

area six

SPLIT MOUNTAIN AND FISH CREEK

6

Many consider the desert dry and desolate but secret oases, cool waterfalls, interesting animals and a wide array of adaptive vegetation wait quietly to refresh adventurous souls

Introduction

Split Mountain Road runs south from CA 78 at Ocotillo Wells, the popular off-road area. The road takes its name from a stream-cut gorge that sliced into what otherwise would have been a solid mountain range. East of the gorge is the Fish Creek Mountains Wilderness Area, controlled by the Bureau of Land Management (BLM) and off-limits to vehicles. The Vallecitos Mountains are to the west.

Spectacular rock formations await you along the dirt route marked "Fish Creek Primitive Camp" off of paved Split Mountain Road. The imposing rock walls tower overhead, with stone peeling away in layers that form circular and diametric patterns. Natural mud caves and hills are also prevalent in this region, making for varied terrain that speaks of the passage of time and environmental changes. Ancient seas once inundated the land here, leaving fossils that now crowd one to the next and layer upon layer.

The large drainage system, Fish Creek Wash, is fed by many smaller washes. Mostly open to (street-legal) vehicles, Fish Creek Wash is often packed with weekenders out in their four-wheel drives. It stretches for many miles through the Vallecitos Mountains, the Carrizo badlands, Split Mountain, and the Lower Borrego Valley. At Split Mountain, squeezing rock walls narrow the wash, which eventually ends east of the Anza-Borrego Desert State Park border in tranquil San Sebastian Marsh.

The area's official camping site is Fish Creek Primitive Camp, but backpacking deeper into the many washes and tributary canyons allows more solitude and peaceful communing with nature. Whether day-hiking or camping, be prepared for temperature changes. Some of the deep washes shadowed by canyon walls can be quite cold, even in warmer weather.

Here I've described hikes ranging from a small taste of the desert aided by a park interpretive guide at Elephant Trees Nature Loop, to much longer treks into remote canyon washes. You'll venture into the shadow of unusual formation "Elephant Knees" to peek at fossils, and ascend to eerie wind caves where the breeze seems to whisper Indian history. From your vantage point, look down at the vast folds and crevices of the Carrizo Badlands. And finally, enjoy moist breezes and pure serenity at San Sebastian Wash.

These hikes are just a few of the possible foot-journeys in the Split Mountain–Fish Creek area. If you're feeling adventurous, a copy of Diana and Lowell Lindsay's *Anza-Borrego Desert Region* map (available at Amazon.com) will help you locate and explore even more.

24 Elephant Trees Nature Loop

SCENERY: ☆☆☆	HIKING TIME: *0.5–1 hour*
DIFFICULTY: ☆	OUTSTANDING FEATURES: *Soft, sandy trail with a few small boulders, views of open sky framed by the Vallecitos Mountains in the distant west, fragrant desert lavender, a variety of cactuses, birds, and jackrabbits*
TRAIL CONDITION: ☆☆☆☆	
SOLITUDE: ☆☆☆	
CHILDREN: ☆☆☆☆☆	
DISTANCE: *1 mile round trip*	

This short loop offers just a sample of desert life. Armed with an interpretive guide found at the trailhead, both novice naturalists and seasoned desert-goers can become mini-experts on the vegetation's survival adaptations in the arid climate and learn how to identify some of the most prevalent native plants.

Grab a nature trail guide from the box at the trailhead and start out southwest along the sandy wash path. This trail is mostly flat, with tiny, hardly noticed elevation gains in spots, making it simple to simultaneously read and walk.

While enjoying views of the Vallecitos Mountains etched against open sky to the west, look around for feathery (but thorny) acacia catclaw growing alongside the trail. In winter months, heavy clumps of desert mistletoe weight the branches. The berries attract the fluttering phainopepla, a small crested bird, to its food source. In the quiet of the trail, you may hear its pleasant one-note call, a constant backdrop in many of the washes in Anza-Borrego Desert State Park.

Desert lavender, with its delicate flowers, is one of the bigger bushes you'll see growing in profusion along the route. The foliage and flowers scent the fresh air with a tangy fragrance as you easily—perhaps even lazily—hike along. The route edges right(northwest) at approximately 0.4 miles and, within a few more yards, passes the halfway mark heading east to begin completing the loop.

The smaller indigo bush also grows here, recognized by narrow gray-green leaves and pale, sometimes white, bark that deflect the

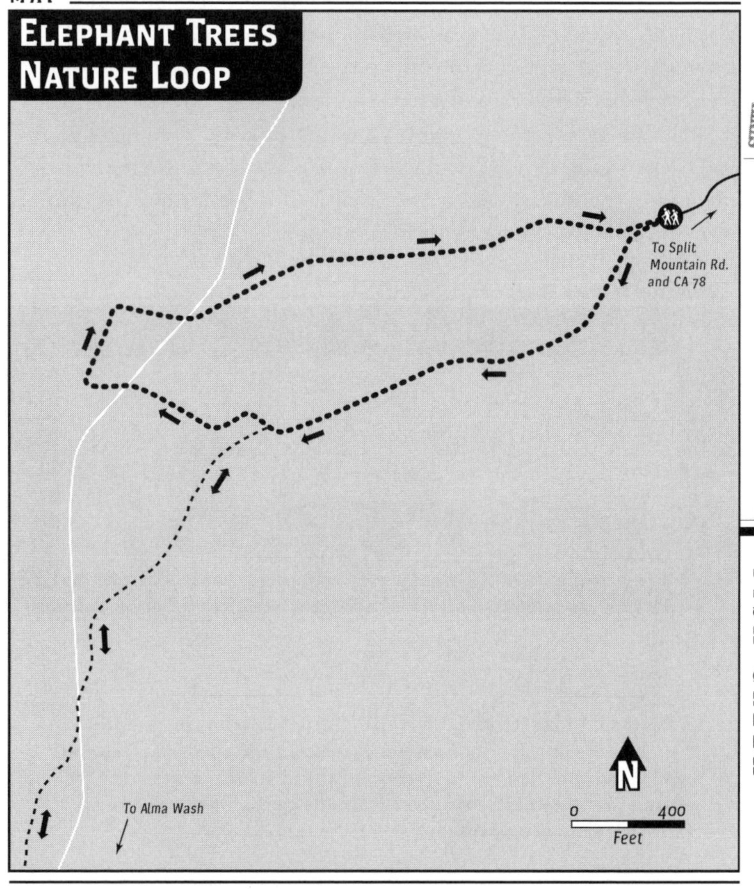

intense sun. Its flowers grow in dark blue-violet indigo torches on the finely branched plant.

The trail is named for the elephant tree, which you'll see here. Although the leaves are small and in no way resemble an elephant's ears, the trees grow 6 to 10 feet tall; twisting branches often spread the tree's width to 15 to 30 feet. In that sense they resemble an elephant, and they also store water in their trunks. The Anza-Borrego Desert region is the only place in California where the trees are considered to be a native species.

Use the trail guide to identify a variety of cacti, then make your way back to your vehicle. As the desert plants adapt to their environment, you should institute a few desert survival techniques of your own—take plenty of water with you on this hike.

ELEVATION PROFILE

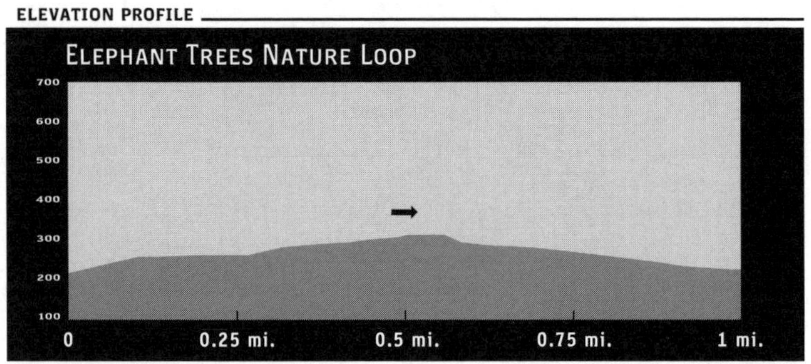

Directions: From CA 78 (at Ocotillo Wells), drive south on Split Mountain Road. After approximately 6 miles, a kiosk marks a rugged, unpaved road. If you are in a truck, or car with higher clearance, you can probably navigate with caution the approximate mile to the trailhead. Otherwise park and walk from there.

GPS Coordinates	24 ELEPHANT TREES NATURE LOOP
UTM Zone (WGS84)	11S
Easting	582454
Northing	3659201
Latitude-Longitude	N 33° 4' 5.7174" W 116° 7' 0.0498"

25 Alma Wash

SCENERY: ☆☆☆
DIFFICULTY: ☆☆☆☆
TRAIL CONDITION: ☆☆
SOLITUDE: ☆☆☆☆☆
CHILDREN: ☆

DISTANCE: *11 miles round trip*
HIKING TIME: *6 hours*
OUTSTANDING FEATURES: *Soft, sandy wash; boulders; cool canyons; and elephant trees*

This long, fairly disused trek offers the gift of silence. The sandy wash gives way to boulders and enters a canyon where the temperature noticeably drops at points where the sun is blocked (wear layers). Long pants and sleeves defend against grabbing catclaw, spiny barrel cactus, and cholla. Careful foot navigation on piled, sometimes-unstable rocks, as well as boulder hopping that increases with mileage covered, make Alma Wash unsuitable for younger, less-experienced hikers. For hardy hikers who enjoy a long, quiet trek into desert solitude, this is the place to find such quiet paradise.

OVERNIGHT OPTION: *Once into the canyon portion of Alma Wash, which leads into the Vallecitos Mountains, the sights and sounds of civilization disappear. Flat areas near the turnaround point make wonderful camping sites.*

Begin at the Elephant Trees Nature Loop trailhead, heading southwest as described on page 140. Then, near signpost marker #6, where the nature trail veers to the right and the wash continues left, head left (southwest). Multitudes of bird and small-animal footprints form a wildlife patina on the powdery sand. You may even see some larger footprints that belong to sheep, coyote, or mountain lions. Fragrant desert lavender frames the wash and becomes your constant companion for nearly the length of this hike.

A little more than 1 mile from the trailhead, the wash moves to the right, heading more directly west but meandering a little, with small, straying flow-fingers forming. Stay on a westerly trek, heading toward a break in the jagged Vallecitos Mountains still more than 2 miles away. As you get closer, the break becomes more defined, a sky-filled U cut

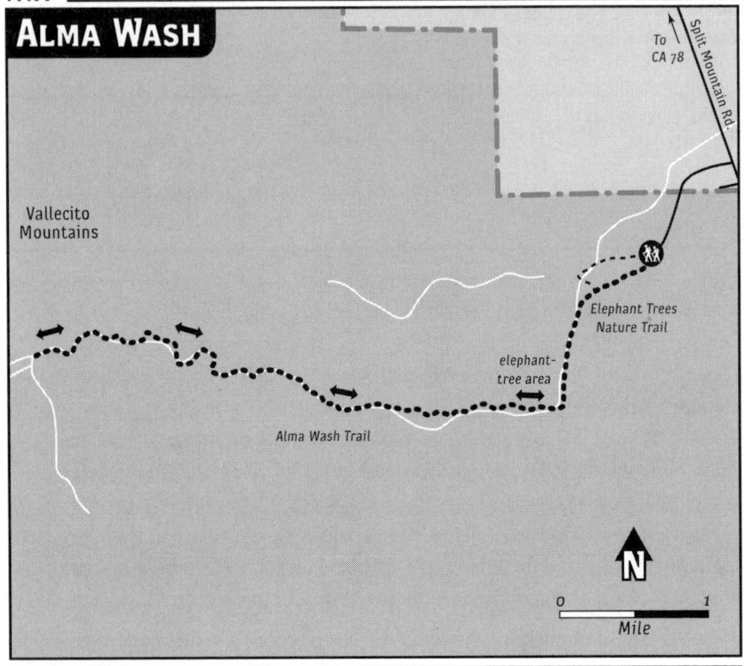

into the mountain silhouette. Either head directly toward it, or follow the wash closely as it meanders, choosing soft sand that sinks with each step or climbing small boulders and dodging fat, spiny barrel cactus—either way is a good leg workout.

Approximately 2.3 miles from the trailhead, you'll begin to see elephant trees, easily identified by their twisting trunks and branches suggestive of an elephant's legs and trunk. The trees have gray bark and red inner flesh and feature small, scented, pinnate-style (feathery) leaves. Native Americans used the elephant tree for medicinal purposes and made the aromatic sap into incense.

At approximately 3 miles, you'll reach the break in the mountains you've been aiming for. The canyon walls rise higher, and the elephant trees disappear for now. Continue up the rocky wash. Boulder hopping becomes the norm as you gain elevation. Be careful moving over piled boulders. Some smaller rocks are unstable and can result in falls. A mile into the canyon, you'll begin again to see elephant trees, most of them clinging to the towering canyon walls. The desert lavender you've begun to take for granted now thins, while rayless daisies (void of the typical ray-type petals) increase. The pollen-rich balls waggle like bobbleheads in the breeze, luring bees to their fertile treasure.

Depending on the position of the sun as it follows its daily pattern from the eastern to western sky, the shadowed canyon can be quite cool—even on warm days. With luck (and preparation!), you've dressed in layers that you can shed and reclaim as the temperature requires.

At about 5.3 miles, thorny catclaw acacia chokes the canyon. Alma Wash seems to split off in every direction into smaller tributaries.

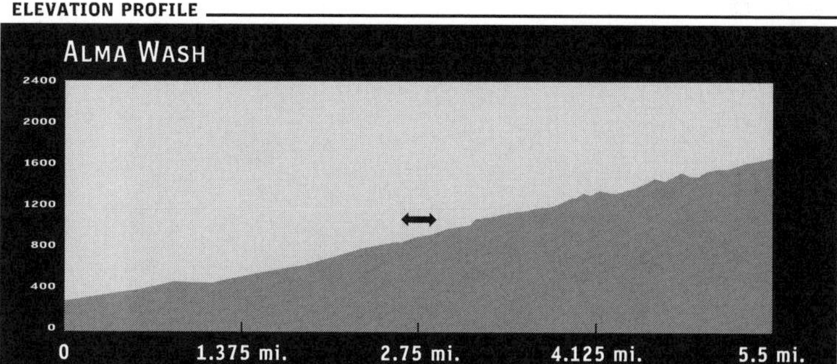

This is a good place to turn around and head back, or perhaps retrace your steps to a good camping spot that you spied on the way.

Whether bedding down for the night in a spot where you can enjoy a blanket of stars unhampered by ambient light, or hiking the whole 5.3 miles back to your car, do take a few moments to enjoy the dense quiet and natural peace within little-visited Alma Wash.

Directions: From CA 78 (at Ocotillo Wells), drive south on Split Mountain Road. After approximately 6 miles, a kiosk marks a rugged, unpaved road. If you are in a truck, or car with higher clearance, you can probably navigate with caution the approximate mile to the trailhead. Otherwise, park and walk from there.

GPS Coordinates	25 ALMA WASH
UTM Zone (WGS84)	11S
Easting	582454
Northing	3659201
Latitude–Longitude	N 33° 4' 5.7174" W 116° 7' 0.0498"

26 Wind Caves Loop

SCENERY: ★★★★	DISTANCE: *1–1.5 miles round trip*
DIFFICULTY: ★★★	HIKING TIME: *1–2 hours*
TRAIL CONDITION: ★★★	OUTSTANDING FEATURES: *Naturally formed hollows and small chambers, and views of the Carrizo badlands*
SOLITUDE: ★★★	
CHILDREN: ★★	

A short, steep trail leads to a series of wind caves once utilized as shelters by Native Americans and offers a viewpoint for overlooking the desert's interesting landscape. Playful hikers can't resist climbing inside a cave or two, perhaps posing for a companion's camera at one of the sand-etched windows in these natural formations.

From the dirt parking area, the narrow trail heads to the right, climbing steeply the first 300 feet, then leveling for a brief breather before resuming the uphill pitch. Though well defined, the path may be slippery due to loose rocks. Tread carefully.

At approximately 0.1 mile, the trail splits. Take either side. The paths merge a short distance ahead. Continue over hills and dales for about 0.33 miles, where the first cave formations come into view on the right. Walk a little farther, venturing into and around the caves as much as your energy and curiosity dictate. Native populations once dwelled in these stooped shelters, setting modern man's mind to wander. Within the cool interiors, sunlight peeks through crevices and naturally formed skylights, making the atmosphere ethereal.

To the left, you'll see a very steep trail. This climbs sharply for 0.25 miles, ending on a sheer precipice overlooking a deep arroyo. If you choose to navigate this steep offshoot trail, be careful. Not only is the path slick, but the edge at the top is so narrow that a gust of wind might send you flying—and wishing you had wings.

To finish the loop, head up through the center area of the cave complex, and access the trail that moves southwest. You'll see another

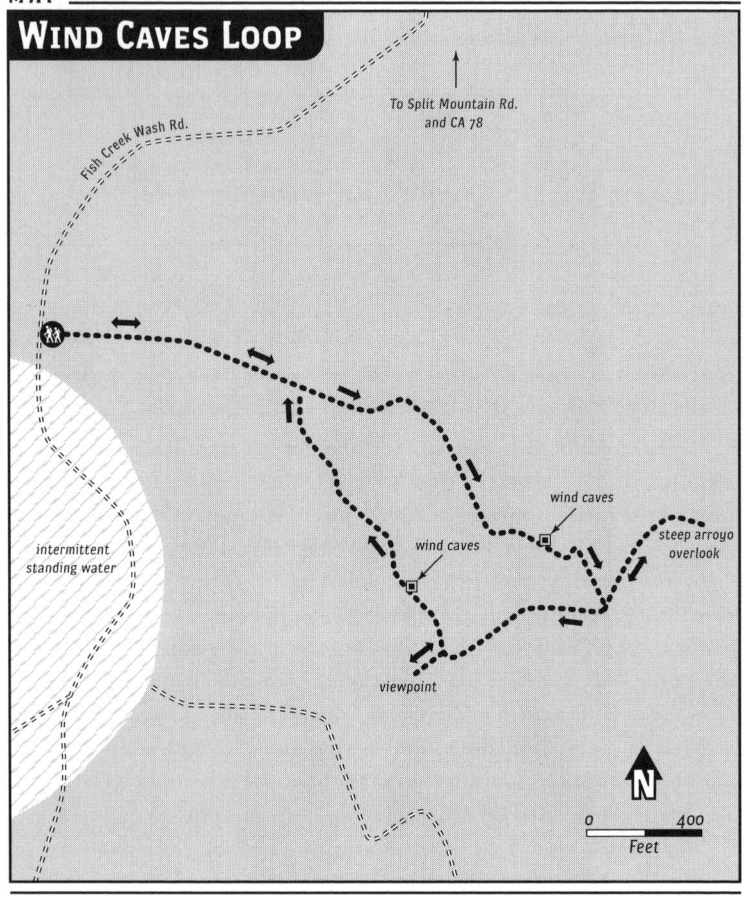
WIND CAVES LOOP
To Split Mountain Rd.
and CA 78
Fish Creek Wash Rd.
wind caves
steep arroyo
overlook
wind caves
intermittent
standing water
viewpoint
N
0
400
Feet

small offshoot trail leading to a safer viewpoint. Perhaps spend a few moments enjoying a wonderful view of the Fish Creek area and the magnificent folds of the Carrizo Badlands, then take the trail down. The undulating route turns northwest and passes even more wind caves on the right before it eventually joins the opening trail. Head left, carefully retracing your steps down the steep section to the bottom.

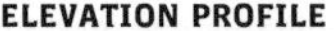

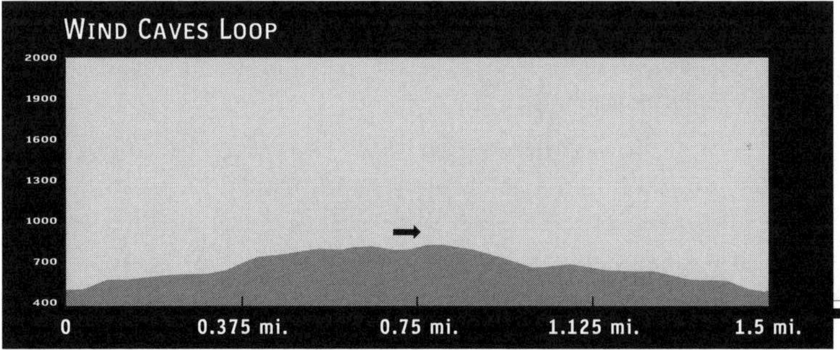

Directions: From CA 78 at Ocotillo Wells, head south on Split Mountain Road for approximately 8 miles. En route, pass the Elephant Trees Nature Loop turnoff (to the right) and continue to another dirt route on the right marked "Fish Creek Wash." Drive up the wash, approximately 5 miles (four-wheel drive recommended), and park on the left, where you will see a small sign marked "Wind Caves."

GPS Coordinates	26 WIND CAVES LOOP
UTM Zone (WGS84)	11S
Easting	582354
Northing	3650874
Latitude–Longitude	N 32° 59' 35.3992"
	W 116° 7' 6.5751"

27 Mud Hills Wash to Elephant Knees

SCENERY: ☆☆☆☆☆	DISTANCE: *4 miles round trip*
DIFFICULTY: ☆	HIKING TIME: *2–3 hours*
TRAIL CONDITION: ☆☆☆☆☆	OUTSTANDING FEATURES: *Mud hills, fossils, typical sandy-wash landscape, and the towering formation known as Elephant Knees*
SOLITUDE: ☆☆☆	
CHILDREN: ☆☆☆☆	

This easy out-and-back trip allows you to view fossils in plain sight, layered like cake in uplifted sandstone buttresses.

Enter the wash beyond the "closed area" sign barring all vehicles and you'll immediately see the aptly named Elephant Knees to the southwest. The shell-reef buttress does in fact look like a series of elephant knees all in a row. The size and configuration is like something out of a *Star Wars* film.

The sandy, mostly level wash moves between hills of mud that sparkle with bits of gypsum gleaming in the sun. In the dull mud, the crystalline gypsum glints like ancient treasure and hints at what's to come—fossils some several millions of years old, remnants of the Gulf of California that at one time covered the area.

The route meanders a little, bending away from Elephant Knees, then back, away and back again. The hulky formation itself will be visible only part of the time beyond the hills of mud bordering the wash. Enjoy the immediate scenery, if not for its beauty, then for its unique qualities. The flaky surface of the dried mud hills holds a rough pattern, similar to elephant skin. An interesting plant found here is the desert trumpet, recognized by a bulging, inflated portion in its central stem. When dry in winter or summer, the perennial upright herb is drab brown with a bulbous stem and spindled head similar to an old television antennae or an invader from Mars. Spring

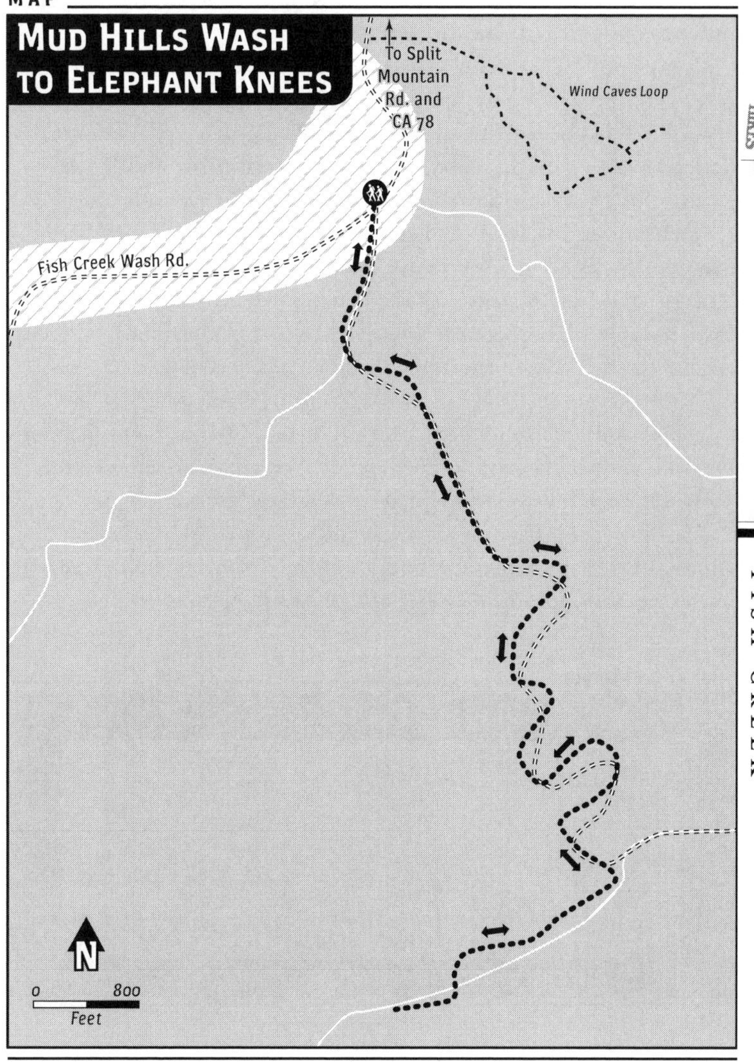

Mud Hills Wash
to Elephant Knees
To Split
Mountain
Rd. and
CA 78
Wind Caves Loop
Fish Creek Wash Rd.
N
0
800
Feet

through early fall, the green spindles sprout small yellow flowers above the trumpet-inflated stem and a spray of flat, green leaves.

At 1.6 miles, the main wash stretches to the left. Turn right here, accessing a narrower side route that quickly bends southwest, heading around the backside of Elephant Knees. The now-rockier path is littered heavily with the glassy gypsum. The trail forks at mile 1.8, paths splitting around some mud domes. Take the right fork.

What do the backs of elephants' knees look like? Saggy and baggy may come to mind, but not in this case. The backside of Elephant Knees is drier and rockier than the buttress front, losing the "knees" form entirely. Here you'll see layers and layers of embedded oyster and shrimp fossils. As you walk along, the fossil presence thickens, seemingly stirred into the land like slivered nuts in cookie dough. There are so many fossils that you'll be walking on them, touching them all along the trail, and seeing them in the distance. Fragments are most common, although fully intact shells are also present en masse.

Visible fossils begin to thin, completely replaced by a more typical desert experience at around 2 miles. Rocky terrain dotted with bushy creosote, spindly ocotillo, and stout barrel cactus seems to

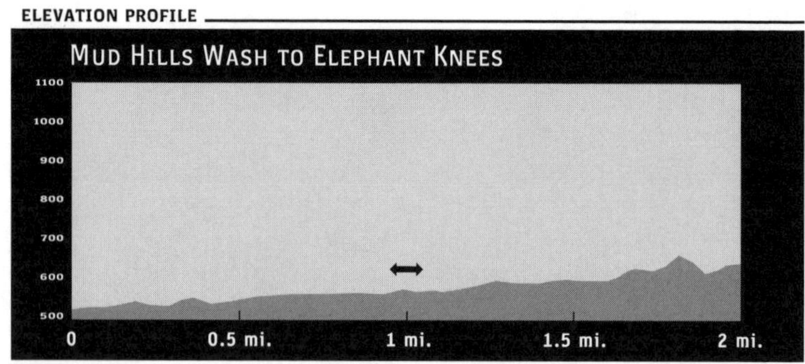

have swallowed the mud hills and fossil-rich landscape—clues to ancient waters once present here and filled with sea life.

Retrace your steps to the main wash, then go left back to Fish Creek Wash, where you've parked. Before leaving, venture up to the kiosk west of the trailhead for a quick study of the Gulf of California while overlooking the rolling mud dunes.

Directions: From CA 78 at Ocotillo Wells, head south on Split Mountain Road for approximately 8 miles. En route, pass the Elephant Trees Nature Loop turnoff (to the right) and continue to another dirt route on the right marked "Fish Creek Wash." Drive up the wash (four-wheel drive recommended). Pass Wind Caves on the left at approximately 5 miles, and bear left (the north fork of Fish Creek Wash splits to the right). Mud Hills Wash is approximately 0.3 miles past the split (unmarked), on the left. You'll recognize it by a sign reading "closed area," barring vehicle use of the wash. Once you see a kiosk (also on the left) with information on the unusual dune formations, you'll have gone too far. Park on the hard sand shoulder, where unmistakable Elephant Knees is visible to the southwest.

GPS Coordinates	27 MUD HILLS WASH TO ELEPHANT KNEES
UTM Zone (WGS84)	11S
Easting	582373
Northing	3650518
Latitude–Longitude	N 32° 59' 23.8121" W 116° 7' 5.9571"

28 San Sebastian Marsh

SCENERY: ☆☆☆	DISTANCE: *4 miles round trip*
DIFFICULTY: ☆	HIKING TIME: *2 hours*
TRAIL CONDITION: ☆☆☆	OUTSTANDING FEATURES: *Soft, sandy wash; water; shells; seabirds; tamarisk; and open desert views*
SOLITUDE: ☆☆☆☆	
CHILDREN: ☆☆☆	

This fairly short hike along the etched channel at the terminus of Fish Creek Wash delivers you from the arid desert air to the refreshingly moist breezes and riparian environment of San Sebastian Marsh. Listed mileage is typical of mid- to late spring, but will vary year-to-year with the weather. The marsh forms where Fish Creek, Carrizo, and San Felipe washes meet.

After parking your vehicle above deep Fish Creek Wash, move on foot down into the gully and begin walking east (left). You may see and hear motorcyclists from nearby Ocotillo Wells, but you'll be heading into BLM land deemed an "Area of Critical Environmental Concern" and therefore off-limits to vehicles. Occasionally, motorcyclists ignore rules, so do be aware of the sound of engines heralding the presence of approaching riders on ATVs.

As you move along the bottom of Fish Creek Wash, hidden from the open desert beyond its sandy walls several feet higher than your head, you'll feel isolated. The din of civilization will ebb, leaving only your thoughts and the rhythmic crunch of sand and dried mud beneath your feet.

In springtime, purple-pink sand verbena dots the landscape with color, often disbursed in clumps. The plants huddle together, forming small communities busy with insects—bees, ants, and beetles. Tamarisk, a non-native tree that's considered invasive and often targeted in San Diego–area removal efforts, also grows here. For the

MAP

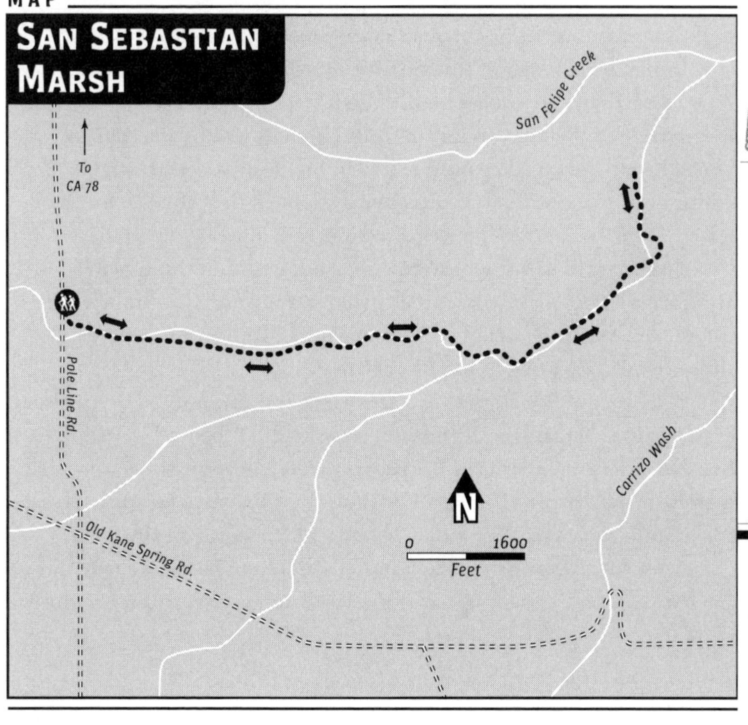

moment, forget its negative status and enjoy the blessings it provides—spots of shade and pretty pink bloom tufts swaying softly in the breeze.

Typically, by mid- to late spring, the first mile of the trek is fairly dry. Baked by the sun, mud dries in puzzle-piece patterns, the topmost layer curling. Beneath your feet, paper-thin surface curls crunch like potato chips. Bigger, thicker mud curls, created where water pooled for longer periods, give way more slowly, their sound like ceramic chimes.

Mud that has dried in stages, creating tissue-thin layers that cling together in an inch-thick group, sound like rumpled cellophane.

In the dense quiet of this sun-dried terrain, listen for subtle nuances, like music you create with each step. Sand, kicked up by wind, frosts some of the dried mud curls, its weight muffling the crunch beneath your feet. Other mud cracks in big, long sheets the shape of continents, while still more pieces curl so much they close in on themselves, forming tubes—all making unique melodies as you tread.

The rhythm of your footsteps may lull you, but don't get too comfortable. The route becomes progressively moister, so be careful where you step. The dried surface may be hiding an underlayer of slippery mud that can send you reeling.

What may at first appear as a frosting of salt in spots is, upon closer examination, actually multitudes of tiny shells left behind as water receded. These remnants of life demonstrate the abundance of water here near the terminus of Fish Creek Wash, which expands or decreases the boundaries of San Sebastian Marsh with changing weather.

After 1.5 miles (or perhaps sooner in wetter years or earlier in the season), small pools of water are likely to appear, often lined with

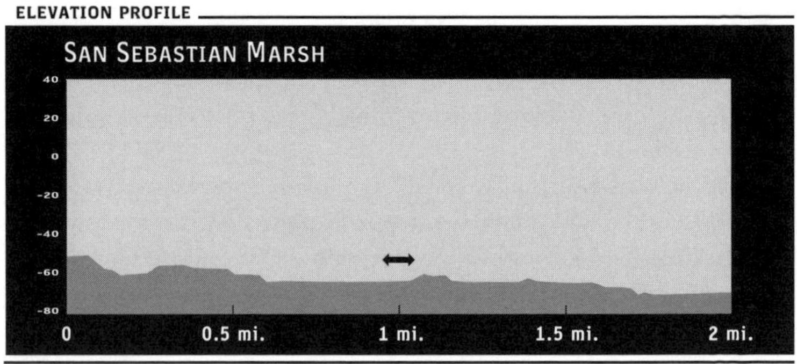

reeds. The air takes on a refreshing quality, infused by moisture that proves the marsh is ahead. You'll begin leaving tracks in the dark mud alongside those of coyote, a variety of birds, and small mammals lured by the life-giving water.

At 2 miles, you'll have likely reached the outskirts of the marsh. Here, you can rest along the water's edge. The glossy surface ripples in the wind. Dragonflies hover and dip. Seabirds wade and peck. Try practicing a Native American version of hunting—quietly sit, allowing nature to resume after the initial disruption of your presence. With patience and silence, wonders await you at San Sebastian Marsh.

Directions: On CA 78, continue east approximately 9 miles past Ocotillo Wells. At the fenced San Felipe Electrical substation, turn right on Pole Line Road (dirt). Continue south, with vehicle-restricted BLM land on either side, for approximately 3.2 miles. Park at the deeply etched Fish Creek Wash.

GPS Coordinates	**28 SAN SEBASTIAN MARSH**
UTM Zone (WGS84)	**11S**
Easting	**595391**
Northing	**3660664**
Latitude–Longitude	**N 33° 4' 49.4108"**
	W 115° 58' 40.6032"

7

area seven

AGUA CALIENTE COUNTY PARK

Many consider the desert dry and desolate but secret oases cool waterfalls interesting animals and a wide array of adaptive vegetation wait quietly to refresh adventurous souls

Introduction

With 140 campsites (many with full hookup service) and two naturally fed hot pools, Agua Caliente County Park is a wonderful place to retreat from the hectic city. Warm showers are available, as is a caravan site for large groups. Located off County Route S2 south of the Vallecitos Mountains, the park is open fall to late spring and closed during the hot summer months. Even just for day use, Agua Caliente County Park provides a safe base point for hiking or picnicking. For fees and additional information, visit **www.co.san-diego.ca.us/parks/camping/agua_caliente.html.**

I've outlined an easy hike, the romantic Moonlight Canyon Loop, which you can access at the south end of the park. From this trail, venture farther into the adjacent washes if you choose. You might also check out the Ocotillo Ridge Nature Trail, which connects to short pond and desert overview routes.

29 Moonlight Canyon Loop

SCENERY: ☆☆☆	DISTANCE: *1.84 miles round trip*
DIFFICULTY: ☆	HIKING TIME: *1 hour*
TRAIL CONDITION: ☆☆☆☆☆	OUTSTANDING FEATURES: *Sandy wash, interesting boulder and erosion formations*
SOLITUDE: ☆☆	
CHILDREN: ☆☆☆☆☆	

The relaxing experience of a brief stroll on an easy trail with a few steep areas and some hops down boulders seems days away from civilization when you take in the quiet. You may see campers out for this stroll at twilight, when the moon begins to rise. Perhaps the short trek is called Moonlight Canyon Loop because it lends itself to friendly chatting as the sun sets.

From the trailhead behind and to the right of the shuffleboard area, you'll begin immediately climbing on the well-worn trail. After about 0.33 miles, you'll reach a side trail that climbs to an elevation of about 1,750 feet—your option. It's a short climb to the peak, which is a good vantage point to the valley.

The trail descends a little, beginning a pattern of rocks underfoot, then sandy wash, rocks, then sand—all rutted into a wide wash path around the peak in the middle. The rocky walls alongside the trail have eroded in intricate patterns, and though this trail is short, there's a sense of isolation. The rock on either side of the path buffers noise, so you may not realize other hikers are near until they are practically upon you.

At about 0.75 miles, the route dips, crossing a wooded seep. You may see birds here, drawn to the water and willows. In fact, Agua Caliente County Park is a well-known spot for birding enthusiasts. You'll find more birds along the pond trail and sometimes even among the individual campsites. Just as alfresco city dining attracts birds, humans picnicking in camping areas also attracts wildlife.

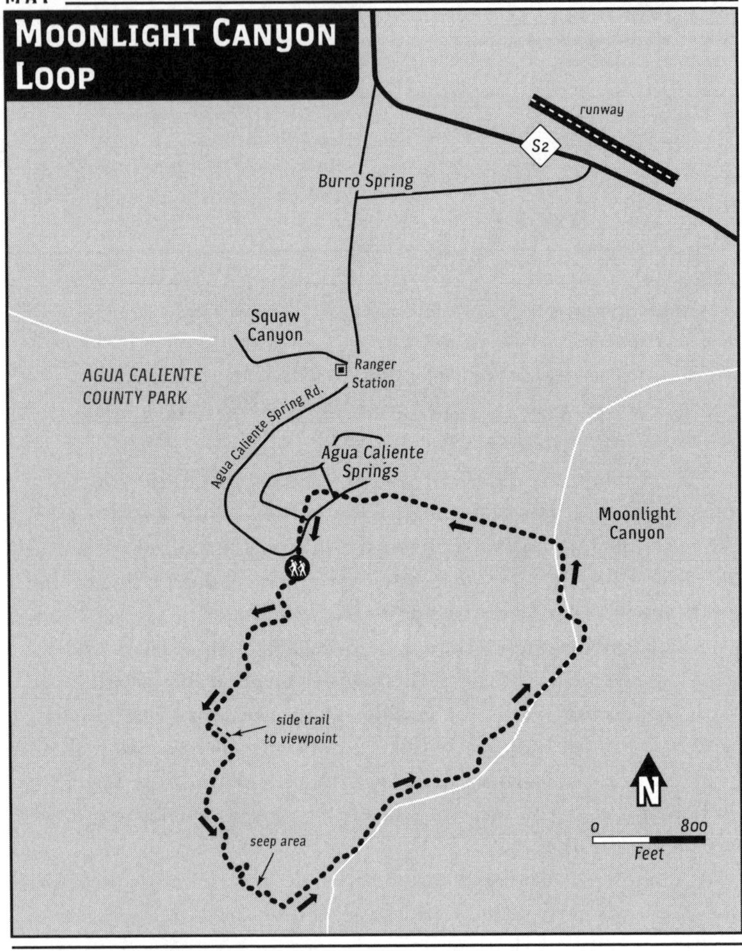

At approximately 1 mile the trail opens up, beginning to make the left curve around the middle peak to close the loop. In the northeast, the Vallecitos Mountains come into view, a formidable ridge in the distance. In late afternoon, the shadows bring out mauves and tans that add an interesting frame to your walk. This peaceful, quiet stretch brings you another 0.4 miles to the campground road, where you'll turn left and follow it back up to your car.

If you've stopped in for a day visit, consider one of the other short trails in the county park, or plan a longer trip back—perhaps with your RV or tent.

ELEVATION PROFILE

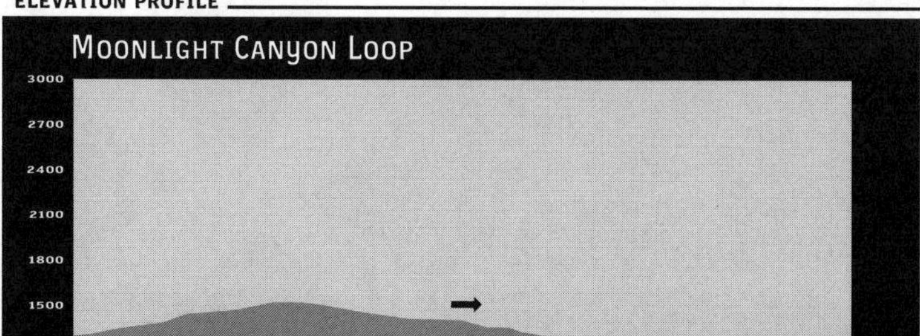

Directions: From Interstate 8E, take the Ocotillo Imperial Highway exit and head northwest on County Route S2. Drive 27 miles to Agua Caliente County Park. Turn left into the park and follow the road southwest to the Ranger Station. You'll pay $5 for day use of any length. The ranger has free maps of the county park's hiking trails. To get to the Moonlight Canyon trailhead, follow the main park road past the mineral pools, and park near the shuffleboard court. The trail begins just right of the court.

GPS Coordinates	29 MOONLIGHT CANYON LOOP
UTM Zone (WGS84)	11S
Easting	565115
Northing	3645798
Latitude–Longitude	N 32° 56' 54.7722"
	W 116° 18' 12.1131"

area eight 8

CARRIZO CREEK AND CARRIZO CANYON

Many consider the desert dry and desolate but secret oases cool waterfalls interesting animals and a wide array of adaptive vegetation wait quietly to refresh adventurous souls

AREA 8: CARRIZO CREEK AND CARRIZO CANYON

Introduction

Carrizo Creek begins in the Inkopah Mountains, streaming down more than 40 miles—northward through Carrizo Gorge and Carrizo Canyon and northeast into the Carrizo Impact Area (previously a bombing site used by the U.S. Army and Navy that is strictly off limits to the public).

Carrizo Canyon is the gap existing between the Jacumba Mountains to the east and the Inkopah Mountains to the west. Venturing into the wide canyon allows views of old San Diego and Arizona Eastern Railroad train trestles to the east, high above the canyon floor. The spectacular trestles are sisters to one of the world's highest wood trestles, built over Goat Canyon, farther south in Carrizo Gorge.

In this region, enjoy the long Carrizo Canyon route to see the trestles, or explore on the north side of County Route S2 by heading into Canyon Sin Nombre. On the outskirts of the Carrizo Badlands, Canyon Sin Nombre offers opportunities for side ventures into slot canyons. Finally, I've included one of my favorite day hikes: a long loop up South Carrizo Creek into Canyon Sin Nombre, then back across S2 into a peaceful stretch of little-used open desert.

On weekends in spring, Canyon Sin Nombre becomes a hot spot for casual camping. You'll see people along the side of the canyon, often with tarps attached to the beds of their four-wheel drives as tents. Turnouts along South Carrizo Creek's decent Jeep road are popular for RVs.

While in the area, you might stop at the Badlands Overlook off S2, adjacent to Canyon Sin Nombre. Especially in the afternoon, when long shadows interplay with the light of a sinking sun, the sculpted earthen folds are a magnificent sight.

30 Carrizo Canyon to Train Trestles

Scenery: ★★★★	Distance: *4–18 miles round trip*
Difficulty: ★★★	Hiking Time: *2–11 hours*
Trail Condition: ★★★★	Outstanding Features: *Sandy wash, interesting rocks, seasonal stream, mortreros, wildlife, and train trestles*
Solitude: ★★★★	
Children: ★★	

If you plan to hike the entire length from County Route S2, you may want to plan an overnight because of the length. But the relatively flat, easy-to-walk terrain makes this trek possible also as an all-day hike. Evidence of illegal immigrants passing through the last 2 miles outlined here may influence your decision about staying overnight—or in choosing a location to camp (probably somewhere in the first 7 miles, where vehicles are allowed). The wide canyon offers solitude, although on busy days you may see people in four-wheel drives before you reach the vehicle closure sign.

OPTIONS: *A four-wheel drive can traverse the first 7 miles, delivering you to the vehicle closure sign, where you can go the last 2 miles on foot—but walking allows you to experience a close-up view of this quiet canyon. You could also park your four-wheel drive somewhere along the route, choosing to hike as many miles as you want.*

From the turnoff on S2, head into the wide canyon, using the flat Jeep road as a general route guide. You'll begin seeing smoke trees almost immediately, recognizable by their gray, smoke-puff appearance from a distance. Tiny deep-blue flowers adorn the thorny trees in spring and summer.

As you move away from S2, the quiet of Carrizo Canyon envelops you. Watch for wildlife in this canyon corridor. On a recent late-spring visit, a troupe of five to seven coyotes trotted silently past, seemingly undisturbed by our presence. Like desert ghosts, the wily pack quickly disappeared into the brush, probably watching the human intruders in their habitat.

MAP

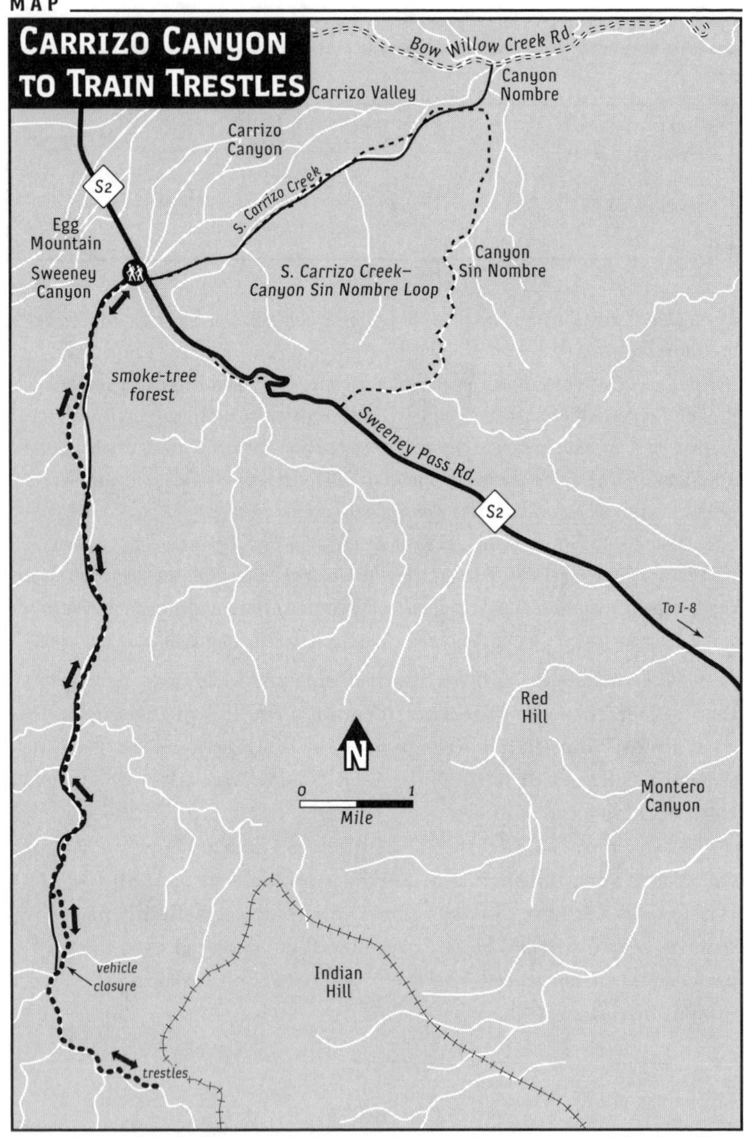

CARRIZO CANYON TO TRAIN TRESTLES
Bow Willow Creek Rd.
Carrizo Valley
Canyon Nombre
Carrizo Canyon
S2
S. Carrizo Creek
Egg Mountain
Sweeney Canyon
Canyon Sin Nombre
S. Carrizo Creek–Canyon Sin Nombre Loop
smoke-tree forest
Sweeney Pass Rd.
S2
To I-8
Red Hill
N
0
1
Mile
Montero Canyon
vehicle closure
Indian Hill
trestles

Delicate tamarisk trees soften the sandy desert-wash landscape. Their delicate pink plumes form a feathery fringe that sways in the breeze. Desert willows also crowd in, evidence of water even when the creek isn't running.

At approximately mile 2.7, Rockhouse Canyon to the west joins Carrizo Canyon. You could cut through here and travel to the old cattleman's rockhouse (see page 126). Continue south on the route that becomes increasingly rock-strewn, giving your legs (or perhaps your four-wheel-drive skills) a workout as you navigate around and over them. At mile 4.3, the east fork of Carrizo Canyon meets the main canyon on the left.

The route meanders, reaching a vehicle closure point at 7 miles. On my last visit, a small compassion station held water and blankets meant for illegal immigrants passing through this region.

From the closure point, a narrower path leads south alongside the creek bed. You'll see mortreros on the rocky east side of the creek. Continuing up the canyon, feathery tamarisk trees encroach on the path, as does spiky acacia catclaw, which also thrives here. At approximately 8.3 miles (1.3 miles past the vehicle closure point), the train trestles become visible above the eastern wall of the canyon. You'll

ELEVATION PROFILE

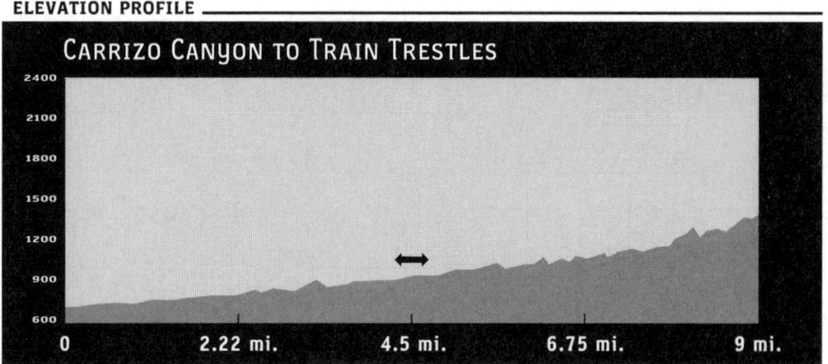

need to cut to the left (east) at this point to avoid thick stands of cat-claw. Climb above the creek bed and continue south. The best views of the trestles occur at approximately 8.5 miles. The route becomes nearly impassable at 9 miles, choked with tamarisk, reeds, and catclaw.

Having seen the trestles, allow yourself to enjoy the scenery on your return trip. Hiking against strong desert winds one recent spring day, I happened upon a hummingbird's nest, securely fastened at eye level in a creosote bush. Inside the minuscule nest cup, a tiny hatchling slumbered next to its still intact sibling egg.

Directions: Where CA 78 meets County Route S2 (the Great Overland Route of 1849), turn right on S2 and head south for 31 miles. En route, you'll see the sign marking your entrance into Anza Borrego Desert State Park at approximately 4.4 miles. After 21 miles, CR S2 veers left (a side road goes straight here, so pay attention). Carrizo Canyon is to the west, a short distance past the sign marking Canyon Sin Nombre to the eastt, and almost directly west of the sign marking Carrizo Creek. Pull off and park.

GPS Coordinates	30 CARRIZO CANYON TO TRAIN TRESTLES
UTM Zone (WGS84)	11S
Easting	574773
Northing	3634663
Latitude–Longitude	N 32° 50' 50.9651" W 116° 12' 3.4377"

31 South Carrizo Creek–Canyon Sin Nombre Loop

Scenery: ☆☆☆☆	Distance: *9.8 miles round trip*
Difficulty: ☆☆☆	Hiking Time: *5 hours*
Trail Condition: ☆☆☆	Outstanding Features: *Sandy wash, open desert, smoke trees, and birds*
Solitude: ☆☆☆	
Children: ☆	

One of my favorite loops, this hike allows you the feel of forging your own path—without having to work too hard at it. The final leg of this trek is on open desert closed to vehicles and not often visited by those on foot. Be alert for surprises. The wild desert never disappoints.

From the parking area (see Directions following), head northeast on the dirt road. The wide-open space is relaxing. Enjoy the vast expanse of the desert beneath a wide sky and framed by rippled mountains in the distance.

After approximately 0.5 miles of easy walking on flat terrain, continue northeast past the strip of pines. The road continues northeast, with creosote bushes becoming the prominent feature (small leaves, yellow blooms, fuzz ball–type fruits). You'll also see some remnants of barbed-wire fencing from Anza-Borrego's cattle days and pass by some turnout spots on the right—probably holding campers on weekends during the busy spring desert-recreation season.

At 3.5 miles, the dirt road comes to a T. Go to the right (east). Vehicle use isn't allowed in this section, so the sandy wash not packed by moving tires becomes looser, making for more difficult walking. After approximately 0.2 miles, the lay of the wash crimps sharply left (southwest). Look due south and notice the V of Canyon Sin Nombre

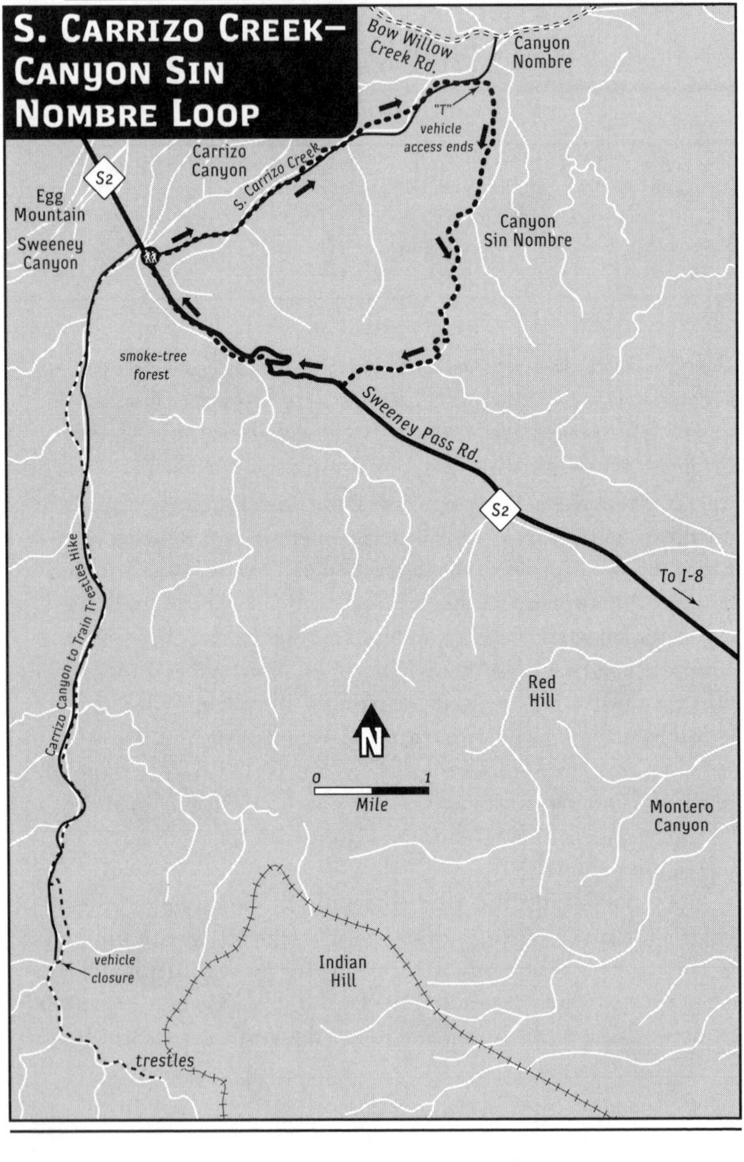

S. Carrizo Creek–Canyon Sin Nombre Loop

Bow Willow Creek Rd.
Canyon Nombre
"T" vehicle access ends
Carrizo Canyon
S. Carrizo Creek
S2
Egg Mountain
Sweeney Canyon
Canyon Sin Nombre
smoke-tree forest
Sweeney Pass Rd.
S2
To I-8
Carrizo Canyon to Train Trestles Hike
Red Hill
N
0
1
Mile
Montero Canyon
Indian Hill
vehicle closure
trestles

ahead. Move away from the main wash, taking a more southerly route to the canyon opening.

Walk south-southwest through Canyon Sin Nombre and follow the vehicle path up to County Route S2 (for details, see Canyon Sin Nombre write-up, page 175). When you reach the highway, you'll have gone 7.4 miles. At S2, turn right and walk on the shoulder, downhill, heading west. After approximately 0.7 miles, you'll approach a hairpin turn of S2. Cross the highway here (careful of any traffic!), and access a trail heading steeply southwest down the ravine (with S2 now on your right). At the bottom, go right, following the northwest bend of the highway. Keep S2 in sight, but there's no need to get too close to the road. Keeping your distance allows you to savor the desolate feel of the open desert.

It's approximately 2 flat miles of sandy wash–type landscape until you spot your vehicle parked on the opposite side of S2. Take your time, enjoying this last, flat leg of the hike. This little-walked area is bound to draw a few stares from passers on the highway. Cars slowing, their inhabitants curious as to what you're doing off the road, is part of the fun. Nature may have a surprise or two as well. On my last visit, I first heard the calls of the logger-head shrike. A few minutes later, what I saw while pausing near

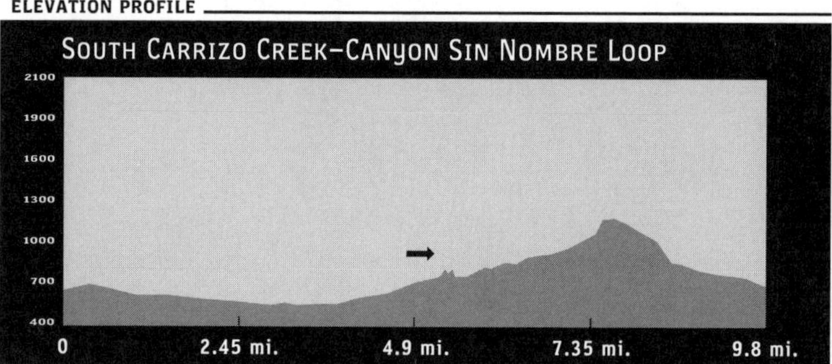

a smoke tree confirmed the birdcall really was that of a loggerhead shrike. Impaled on the thorn of a smoke tree hung the proof—a decapitated lizard. Nicknamed the butcherbird for its habit of hanging its prey from barbed wire or thorns, the loggerhead shrike doesn't have the strong talons of other predator birds. Therefore, it uses this impaling technique to compensate, allowing it to shred the kill into bite-sized pieces.

Directions: From Interstate 8E, take the Ocotillo Imperial Highway exit and head northwest on County Route S2 (the Great Overland Route of 1849). Drive 12.8 miles, just past the Canyon Sin Nombre turnout, to the sign marker for South Carrizo Creek, also on the right. As an alternative, where CA 78 meets CR S2, head south on CR S2 for approximately 32 miles. En route, you'll see the sign marking your entrance into Anza-Borrego Desert State Park at about 4.4 miles. After 21 miles, CR S2 veers left (a side road goes straight here, so pay attention). The Carrizo Creek turnoff is on the left. Park just off the Jeep road (so others can pass), near S2.

GPS Coordinates	31 SOUTH CARRIZO CREEK—CANYON SIN NOMBRE LOOP
UTM Zone (WGS84)	11S
Easting	574945
Northing	3634464
Latitude–Longitude	N 32° 50' 44.4583" W 116° 11' 56.8682"

32 Canyon Sin Nombre

SCENERY: ☆☆☆	DISTANCE: *6 miles round trip*
DIFFICULTY: ☆☆	HIKING TIME: *2.5–3 hours*
TRAIL CONDITION: ☆☆☆☆☆	OUTSTANDING FEATURES: *Sandy wash, slot canyons, smoke trees, and birds*
SOLITUDE: ☆☆	
CHILDREN: ☆☆☆☆☆	

A rather brief jaunt into the canyon cut by floodwaters allows for glimpses of interesting geological characteristics and eroded sandstone formations. Since Canyon Sin Nombre serves as a vehicle throughway to and from Carrizo Creek, you may see four-wheel drives. Traffic may be heavy on weekends (especially in spring), when entire cavalcades forge through the land. You'll likely also see people camping in Canyon Sin Nombre.

From the parking turnoff, head down the wide, well-trodden vehicle route (soft sand) that moves northeast. Gravity is on your side for nearly the whole first mile, but don't go too fast to smell the proverbial roses. Allow the spindly, red-bloomed ocotillos, the stout barrel cactus, and the soft calls of flitting birds to transform your nature trek into magic.

At 1 mile, you'll turn left into the canyon opening, almost immediately wowed by the layered walls of metamorphic rock. The stone forms a rather narrow corridor of sorts, widening out after approximately 0.25 miles.

In spring, notice the pale-purple aster flowers cascading down the canyon walls. Gray-green smoke trees are also prevalent. Watch for another interesting form of vegetation found in Canyon Sin Nombre—the stalked puffball. It is the desert's adaptation to similar fungi from cooler climates. The stalk holds the elongated oval ball up off the hot desert sand, protecting the spores inside from overheating. Under opportune conditions, the ball bursts, releasing an inky cloud of fertile spores on the wind.

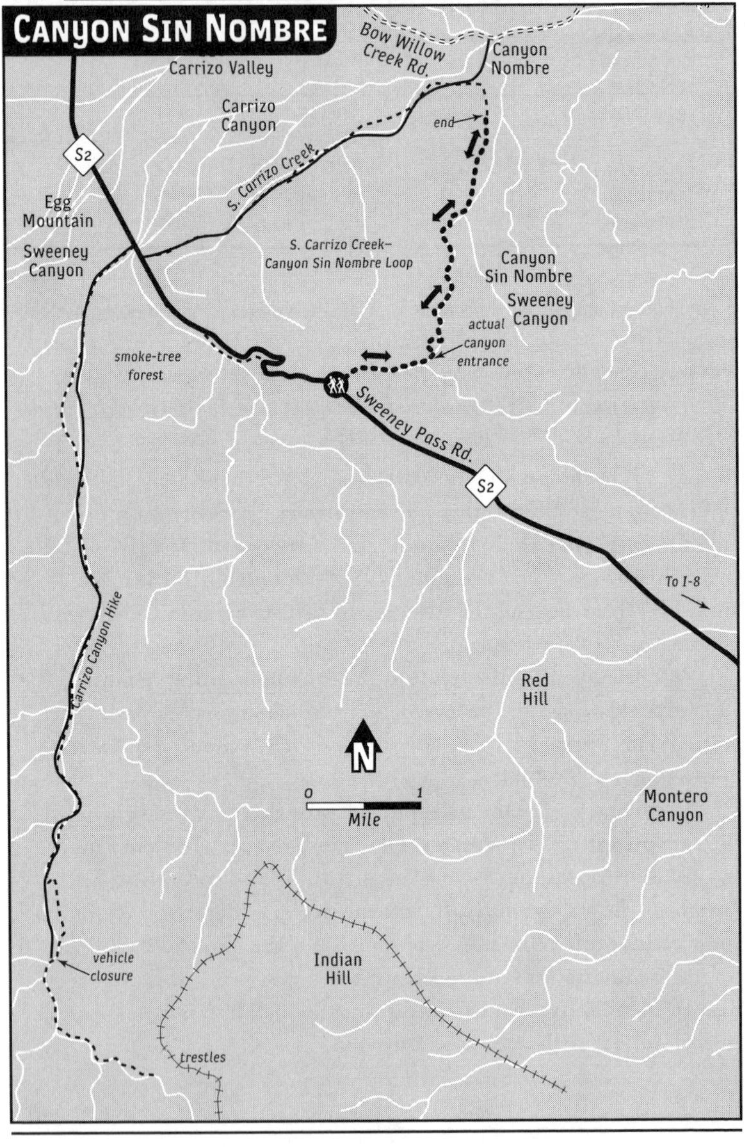

Canyon Sin Nombre

Bow Willow Creek Rd.
Canyon Nombre
Carrizo Valley
Carrizo Canyon
end
S. Carrizo Creek
S2
Egg Mountain
Sweeney Canyon
S. Carrizo Creek– Canyon Sin Nombre Loop
Canyon Sin Nombre
Sweeney Canyon
actual canyon entrance
smoke-tree forest
Sweeney Pass Rd.
S2
To I-8
Carrizo Canyon Hike
Red Hill
N
0
1
Mile
Montero Canyon
Indian Hill
vehicle closure
trestles

At about 1.5 miles, a narrow slot canyon opens on the west side. If you have the time and energy, use the side route to explore, marveling at the slots with towering walls through which you'll squeeze.

The canyon ends, opening into flat wash land, at around 2.5 miles. This is a good turnaround point for a short day hike.

ELEVATION PROFILE

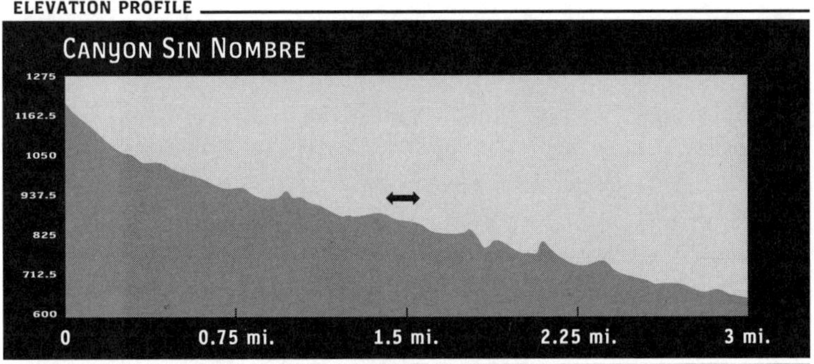

Directions: From Interstate 8E, take the Ocotillo Imperial Highway exit and head northwest on County Rouse S2 (the Great Overland Route of 1849). Drive 12.8 miles to the Canyon Sin Nombre turnout parking area on the right. As an alternative, where CA 78 meets CR S2, head south on CR S2 for approximately 32 miles. En route, you'll see the sign marking your entrance into Anza-Borrego Desert State Park at approximately 4.4 miles. After 21 miles, CR S2 veers left (a side road goes straight here, so pay attention). The Canyon Sin Nombre turnoff is on the left.

GPS Coordinates	32 CANYON SIN NOMBRE
UTM Zone (WGS84)	11S
Easting	577669
Northing	3632779
Latitude–Longitude	N 32° 49' 49.0898"
	W 116° 10' 12.5874"

Appendix A—Outdoor Shops

Adventure 16

www.adventure16.com

2002 South Coast Highway
Oceanside, CA 92054
(760) 966-1700

4620 Alvarado Canyon Road
San Diego, CA 92120
(619) 283-2374

143 South Cedros Avenue
Solana Beach, CA 92075
(858) 755-7662

4348 Convoy Street
San Diego, CA 92111
(858) 560-0311

666 Fletcher Parkway
San Diego, CA 92120
(619) 444-8139

3729 Rosecrans Street
San Diego, CA 92110
(619) 298-3350

760 Sycamore Avenue
Vista, CA 92083
(760) 727-2859

6061-A El Cajon Boulevard
San Diego, CA 92115
(619) 583-7930

2301 Vista Way
Oceanside, CA 92054
(760) 757-4154

Bargain Center Surplus

3015 North Park Way
San Diego, CA 92104
(619) 295-1181

Big 5 Sporting Goods

www.big5sportinggoods.com

1253 East Valley Parkway
Escondido, CA 92027
(760) 480-6860

949 Lomas Santa Fe Drive
Solana Beach CA 92075
(858) 755-5953

8145 Mira Mesa Boulevard
San Diego, CA 92126
(858) 693-4941

16773-B Bernardo Center Drive
Rancho Bernardo, CA 92128
(858) 673-9219

C&C Outdoors

www.ccoutdoorstore.com

3231 Sports Arena Boulevard, Suite 104
San Diego, CA 92110
(619) 222-2326
(888) 385-3456

Cal Stores

1019 Garnet Avenue
San Diego, CA 92109

4030 Sports Arena Boulevard
San Diego, CA 92110

GI Joes Army & Navy Surplus

544 Sixth Avenue
San Diego, CA 92111
(619) 531-1910

REI

www.rei.com
2015 Birch Road, Suite 150
Chula Vista, CA 91915
(opens October 2006)

1590 Leucadia Boulevard
Encinitas, CA 92024
(760) 944-9020

1640 Camino Del Rio North
San Diego, CA 92108
(619) 718-7070

5556 Copley Drive
San Diego, CA 92111
(858) 279-4400

Sport Chalet

www.sportchalet.com
3695 Midway Drive
San Diego, CA 92110
(619) 224-6777

1640 Camino Del Rio North
San Diego, CA 92108
(619) 718-7070

4545 La Jolla Village Drive
San Diego, CA 92122
(858) 453-5656

Sportmart

www.sportmart.com
5500 Grossmont Center Drive
La Mesa, CA 91942
(619) 697-8160

7725 Balboa Avenue
San Diego, CA 92111
(858) 292-0800

11690 Carmel Mountain Road
San Diego, CA 92128
(858) 673-9700

Sports Authority

www.thesportsauthority.com
390 East H Street
Chula Vista, CA 91910

1050 North El Camino Real
Encinitas CA 92024
(760) 634-6690

1352 West Valley Parkway
Escondido, CA 92029
(760) 735-8501

2160 Vista Way
Oceanside, CA 92054
(760) 967-1891

8550 Rio San Diego Drive
San Diego, CA 92108
(619) 295-1682

Appendix B—Places to Buy Maps

Adventure 16

www.adventure16.com
2002 South Coast Highway
Oceanside, CA 92054
(760) 966-1700

4620 Alvarado Canyon Road
San Diego, CA 92120
(619) 283-2374

143 South Cedros Avenue
Solana Beach, CA 92075
(858) 755-7662

C&C Outdoors

www.ccoutdoorstore.com
3231 Sports Arena Boulevard, Suite 104
San Diego, CA
(619) 222-2326, (888) 385-3456

Map Centre

3191 Sports Arena Boulevard
San Diego, CA 92110
(619) 291-3830

REI

www.rei.com
(See facing page for San Diego–area store locations.)

Appendix C—Hiking Clubs and Organizations

BACK COUNTRY LAND TRUST OF SAN DIEGO COUNTY
www.bclt.org
338 West Lexington Avenue, Suite 204
El Cajon, CA 92020
(619) 590-2258

ENCINITAS TRAILS COALITION
www.encinitastrails.org/join
330 Rosemary Lane
Olivenhain, CA 92024

FALLBROOK LAND CONSERVANCY
www.sdlcc.org/flc
P.O. Box 2701
Fallbrook, CA 92028-2701
(760) 728-0889

SAN DIEGO NATURAL HISTORY MUSEUM'S "CANYONEERS"
www.sdnhm.org/canyoneers
P.O. Box 121390
San Diego, CA 92112-1390
(619) 255-0425

SAN DIEGO SEA TO SEA TRAIL FOUNDATION
www.seatoseatrail.org
P.O. Box 19413
San Diego, CA 92159-0413
(619) 303 6975

SIERRA CLUB, SAN DIEGO CHAPTER
sandiego.sierraclub.org/home/index.asp
3820 Ray Street
San Diego, CA 92104
(619) 299-1744

SAN ELIJO LAGOON CONSERVANCY
www.sanelijo.org
P.O. Box 230634
Encinitas, CA 92023
(760) 436-3944

WALKABOUT INTERNATIONAL
4639 30th Street, Suite C
San Diego, CA 92116

Index

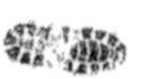

I

J

K

L

M

N

O

About the Author

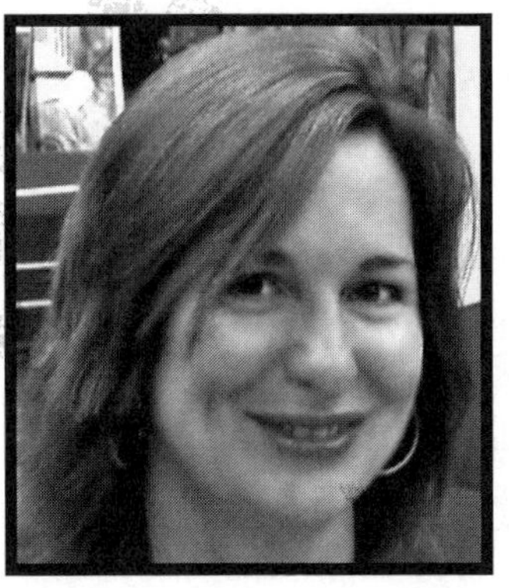

As a child growing up in San Diego, Sheri McGregor remembers lying in the grass watching tiny bug worlds crawl by. Today, with five children of her own, she still watches bugs . . . and sometimes feels just as tiny among the towering trees, majestic mountains, and free-flowing waters of San Diego and adjacent counties. Authoring hiking guides allows Sheri to share her love of the local wilderness, where even the shadows fall into intricate patterns that display the poetry of nature. For hikes closer to the city, consult her *60 Hikes within 60 Miles: San Diego* (Menasha Ridge Press).

In addition to writing about nature and the outdoors, Sheri has published two novels and a novella and writes about a variety of subjects, from psychology and fitness to travel and home décor. Her nonfiction articles, short fiction, and memoir have appeared in themed anthologies, a supplemental textbook, and national and international publications including Salon.com, the *Washington Post, InfoWeek, LA Parent, San Jose, Sunset,* and *Walking.* She also assists with companies' communication and marketing needs and writes for such nonprofit organizations as the Massachusetts-based Families for Depression Awareness.

Visit and write to Sheri at **www.sandiegohikes.com**.

Other Books in This Series

Day and Overnight Hikes: Great Smoky Mountains National Park

Day and Overnight Hikes: Kentucky's Sheltowee Trace

Day and Overnight Hikes: Oregon's Pacific Crest Trail

Day and Overnight Hikes: Shenandoah National Park

Day and Overnight Hikes: West Virginia's Monongahela National Forest

Day and Section Hikes: The John Muir Trail

Visit **www.menasharidge.com** for the full skinny on all the latest Menasha Ridge Press how-to and where-to outdoor guidebooks:

Hiking, backpacking, camping, paddling, mountain biking, road biking, climbing, walking survival, cookbooks, medical guides, fire craft, navigation, and more . . .

Also visit Sheri McGregor's blog site at **www.trekalong.com.** There you can keep current with trail updates, new trails, and author events, and become a member of the *Day and Overnight Hikes* community by blogging along with the author.

Have feedback about this book? E-mail the author at mcgregor@ trekalong.com.